D0874392

The Little Book
of
MENOPA SE

Living with the Challenges
of Breast Cancer

James R. Woods, Jr., M.D.

Elizabeth Warner, M.D.

Adrienne Bonham, M.D.

ABOUT THE AUTHORS

James R. Woods, Jr., M.D. is Professor and past Chairman of the Department of Obstetrics and Gynecology at the University of Rochester School of Medicine and Dentistry in Rochester, New York. Dr. Woods has authored or co-authored over one hundred forty articles on communication in medicine, maternal drug addiction, complications of pregnancy, menopause management, and clinical research. Since 1991, he has been the editor-in-chief of the periFACTS® OB/GYN Academy, an international online educational program for obstetric and gynecologic care providers combining articles, clinical cases, grand rounds lectures, and teaching videos. In 1996, an endowed chair honoring Dr. Woods was established at the University of Rochester. He has been named in Best Doctors in America for many years. In 2010, Dr. Woods was honored by the American College of Obstetricians and Gynecologists with the Outstanding Service Award for District II for his "tireless efforts in the area of obstetric patient safety." In 2012, he received the lifetime achievement award from the District II American College of Obstetricians and Gynecologists. In 2017, Dr. Woods and Dr. Elizabeth Warner published their first menopause book entitled The *Little Book of Menopause; Essays on the Biology and Management of Menopause*. Dr. Woods has lectured extensively on communication in obstetrics and gynecology. He has pioneered strategies for transforming some of the most challenging clinical interactions with patients into extraordinary opportunities for compassionate communication between clinicians and their patients and family members.

Elizabeth D. Warner, M.D. received her undergraduate degree with honors from Cornell University (CALS) in 1975 and her medical degree from the University of Rochester School of Medicine and Dentistry (URMC), M.D. in 1979, member of Alpha Omega Alpha. She was a resident in the University of Rochester Strong Memorial Hospital Obstetrics and Gynecology program from 1979 to 1983. In August of 1983, she joined a private practice in Rochester, New York from which she retired in June of 2013. For approximately 20 years, she was the managing physician of this practice, and for the last ten years of her practice she had a particular interest in menopausal medicine. While in private practice, she held a teaching appointment at the University of Rochester Medical Center. She is currently Clinical Emeritus Professor of Obstetrics and Gynecology, and she continues to teach medical students. She also has an interest in editing, and she is an active medical editor of periFACTS®, an online continuing education program for obstetric and gynecologic care providers. She is a Fellow of the American College of Obstetricians and Gynecologists (ACOG) and a member of the North American Menopause Society (NAMS), the American Society of Colposcopy and Cervical Pathology (ASCCP), and the American Urogynecologic Society (AUGS). She is married to a corporate healthcare attorney, now retired, and has adult identical twin sons.

Adrienne D. Bonham, M.D., M.S. is an Associate Professor and the current Associate Chair for Clinical Affairs and Chief of General Obstetrics and Gynecology at the University of Rochester. She obtained her medical degree from the State University of New York at Buffalo where she was inducted into the Alpha Omega Alpha medical honor society, and completed her residency in Obstetrics and Gynecology at the University of Rochester. She also has a Master's of Science Degree from the University of Pittsburgh School of

Public Health in human genetics and genetic counseling and a Master's of Science Degree in Medical Management from the University of Rochester's Simon School of Business, where she was inducted into the Beta Gamma Sigma business school honor society. Following residency, she worked in a private practice setting for three years before taking on an academic practice where she was the Medical Director for the hospital's clinic for underserved women. She currently specializes in the field of lower genital tract disorders and has a primarily referral-based practice with a catchment area that includes most of Upstate New York and Northern Pennsylvania. She is actively involved in the teaching of both medical students and residents and is the Director of the Division of General Obstetrics and Gynecology at the University of Rochester. Her areas of research interest include vulvovaginal disorders and painful intercourse. She is a member of the North American Menopause Society (NAMS) and is a NAMS-Certified Menopause Practitioner. She is also a Fellow of the American College of Obstetricians and Gynecologists (ACOG), a member of the American Society of Colposcopy and Cervical Pathology (ASCCP), a member of the Society for Academic Specialists in General Obstetrics and Genecology (SASGOG) and has been inducted as a Fellow in the International Society for the Study of Vulvovaginal Disease (ISSVD).

CONTRIBUTORS

Ashley N. Amalfi, M.D.
Assistant Professor
Department of Plastic Surgery
University of Rochester Medical Center
Rochester, New York

Katrina Blackburn Mitchell, M.D.
Clinical Assistant Professor
Department of Surgery
University of New Mexico
Albuquerque, New Mexico

Adrienne D. Bonham, M.D., M.S.
Associate Professor
Department of Obstetrics & Gynecology
University of Rochester Medical Center
Rochester, New York

Elaina Y. Chen, M.D.
Resident
Department of Plastic Surgery
University of Rochester Medical Center
Rochester, New York

Hester Hill-Schnipper, L.I.C.S.W., BCD, OSW-C
Program Manager, Oncology Social Work
Beth Israel Deaconess Medical Center
Boston, Massachusetts

Alissa J. Huston, M.D.
Associate Professor
Department of Hematology/Oncology
University of Rochester Medical Center
Rochester, New York

Michelle Janelsins, Ph.D., M.P.H.
Associate Professor
Department of Surgery, Cancer Control
University of Rochester Medical Center
Rochester, New York

Jayne E. Knowlton, M.S. O.T.R./L.
Department of Physical Medicine and
Rehabilitation/Occupational Therapy
University of Rochester Medical Center
Rochester, New York

Po-Ju Lin, Ph.D., M.P.H., R.D.
Postdoctoral Associate
Department of Surgery, Cancer Control
University of Rochester Medical Center
Rochester, New York

Allison M. Magnuson, D.O.
Assistant Professor
Department of Hematology/Oncology
University of Rochester Medical Center
Rochester, New York

Shirley S. Mandeville, F.N.P., B.C.
Nurse Practitioner
University of Rochester Medical Center
Rochester, New York

Michael T. Milano, M.D., Ph.D.
Associate Professor
Department of Radiation Oncology
University of Rochester Medical Center
Rochester, New York

Kelly Q. Minks, M.S.
Assistant, Department of Genetics
University of Rochester Medical Center
Rochester, New York

Karen M. Mustian, Ph.D., M.P.H.
Professor
Department of Surgery, Cancer Control
University of Rochester Medical Center
Rochester, New York

Edward R. Newton, M.D., F.B.A.M.
Emeritus Professor
Department of Obstetrics and Gynecology
Brody School of Medicine
East Carolina University
Greenville, North Carolina

Avice M. O'Connell, M.D., F.A.C.R.
Professor
Department of Imaging Sciences
University of Rochester Medical Center
Rochester, New York

Thomas D. Rodgers, Jr., M.D.
Department of Hematology/Oncology
James P. Wilmot Cancer Institute
University of Rochester Medical Center
Rochester, New York

Lidia Schapira, M.D., F.A.S.C.O.
Associate Professor
Department of Medicine
Stanford University School of Medicine
Stanford, California

CONTRIBUTORS (CONT.)

Audrey L. Schroeder, M.S.
Assistant
Department of Genetics
University of Rochester Medical Center
Rochester, New York

Michelle Shayne, M.D.
Associate Professor
Department of Hematology/Oncology
University of Rochester Medical Center
Rochester, New York

Manisha P. Sheth O.T.D., O.T.R./L.
Occupational Therapist
Stamford, Connecticut

Wendy S. Vitek, M.D.
Associate Professor
Department of Obstetrics and Gynecology
University of Rochester Medical Center
Rochester, New York

Elizabeth Driggs Warner, M.D.
Clinical Professor Emeritus
Department of Obstetrics & Gynecology
University of Rochester Medical Center
Rochester, New York

Frances Wong, M.D.
Cancer and Hematology Centers of Western
Michigan, P.C.
Grand Rapids, Michigan

James R. Woods, Jr., M.D.
Professor
Department of Obstetrics and Gynecology
University of Rochester Medical Center
Rochester, New York

CONTENTS

PREFACE

Menopause management now is an evidence-based, structured, and formal aspect of medicine. Based upon ongoing research and clinical education from the North American Menopause Society and the American College of Obstetricians and Gynecologists, practice protocols now are able to address the care of women who are either entering menopause (the menopause transition) or are in menopause. Unfortunately, for many women, the diagnosis of breast cancer creates many obstacles to menopause management leading patients to seek advice from their gynecologists. New insights into these cancer-related questions, however, allow gynecologists to understand these concerns and serve as part of the cancer-care team. In this latest contribution to our Little Book of Menopause series, brief discussions and extended discussions by members of the cancer care team address these questions.

Where does communication between care provider and patient break down? The trauma of being diagnosed with breast cancer is amplified if the surgeon, oncologist, and radiologist-oncologist complete their work but fail to address menopausal care. These women struggle with hot flashes, mood swings, pain on intercourse, depression, and marital conflict, but when seeking professional help, they often are confronted by the phrase "no hormones for you."

Most women, especially menopausal women, struggle with questions about breast cancer. How should I be screened? Is genetic counseling important for me and my family? What is the relationship of estrogen to breast cancer? And why is breast cancer divided into types, and for what purpose?

Apart from those women who are made anxious about the general topic itself, becoming a breast cancer survivor often involves menopause. Yet, every woman experiencing breast cancer care that is complicated by menopausal symptoms only wants to feel normal. She asks how to be treated for menopausal symptoms. She also may be haunted by concerns about the psychology of living with breast cancer, the role of her partner, her response to lymphedema and cognitive impairment (chemobrain), her need for exercise, and the challenge of sleep. Or, she may want clarification of how to preserve her reproductive capabilities during treatments, risks of a pregnancy after breast cancer, and whether breastfeeding is possible.

We hope that care providers will find this Little Book contribution to the breast cancer literature a useful resource for their office and for their patients.

BRIEF DISCUSSIONS
UNDERSTANDING MENOPAUSE
(AT THE MOST BASIC LEVEL)

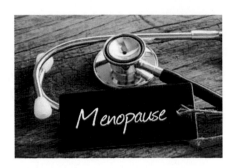

Recent advances in the biology of menopause have helped clarify the importance of female hormones in women's overall health. Improved patient education that allows women to engage in formal conversations with their care providers helps clinicians to individualize menopause management for their patients. In essence, while menopause is a complex process, it can be understood at a basic level by viewing it simply as a process of hormone withdrawal. And the hormone of most importance is estradiol, cyclically produced in large amounts by the ovaries during the reproductive years, reflecting the high numbers of eggs that rapidly decrease in number as one approaches menopause.

During reproductive years, estradiol is critical for menstrual cycles and pregnancy. More recently, scientists have found that during these years, estradiol also has an anti-inflammatory action, preventing immune cells and visceral fat cells from activating certain inflammatory cytokines, including interleukin 1, interleukin 6 and tumor necrosis factor alpha. Yet, it is these same inflammatory proteins that our scientists have linked to essentially all of the more common menopausal symptoms, such as hot flashes, mood swings, memory loss, dry skin, vaginal dryness, low libido, bone breakdown, and cardiovascular risk.

In the past, menopause was considered one full year without any menstruation. We now know that in the several months-to-years leading up to that one year without menstruation, the ovaries gradually become more resistant to hormone control from the brain. This window in time, previously known as perimenopause, now is formally termed the Menopause Transition. Women may only recognize

1

this by encountering irregular menstrual periods. During this interval, however, fluctuations of estradiol from the ovaries begin to allow immune cells and visceral fat cells to release low levels of these inflammatory cytokines into the bloodstream. The result is that these women may begin to experience early menopause symptoms, even though they still are having irregular periods.

The menopause transition represents more than simply the emergence of early menopausal symptoms. This period is associated with significant increases in visceral fat, cholesterol and triglycerides; thickening of the walls of carotid arteries; weight gain; and reduced physical activity.

During menopause, estradiol essentially becomes undetectable in the blood. One would expect that all women, therefore, would experience the classic symptoms of menopause, but that is not so. Despite low levels of estradiol, women entering menopause will differ in how they perceive absence of estradiol. Some will experience only minimal or mild symptoms, while others will feel that they are overwhelmed by new, distressing symptoms. The duration of these symptoms also differs among women. For some women, symptoms will pass within a few years. Recent longitudinal studies now indicate that for other women, symptoms of menopause may last well into their 60s or even 70s.

Scientists have helped clarify the biology of menopause. Clinicians now better understand the range of responses women experience during menopause. These two revelations have matured the field of menopause medicine. Some women will find that education alone is sufficient. Others will need the education to enter into a conversation regarding management. Whether it is through therapeutic listening, complementary and alternative medicines, or hormone replacement, menopause medicine now is a rich, mature, and established field of medicine. Women have always known that menopause is real. The medical community still is working to improve each woman's menopausal life.

MENOPAUSE OR MENOPAUSE TRANSITION: WHEN DOES THE BIOLOGY BEGIN?

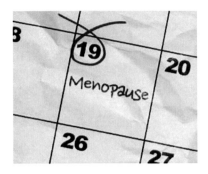

Does menopause really begin only after a woman experiences her last menstrual period? On average, the age of these women is 51 years. But ask any woman in menopause how she recalls the three to five years before she reached that milestone and most will remember that their menstrual cycles became more erratic and unpredictable. We now know that other biological changes also are beginning to occur.

The official statement of the North American Menopause Society (2012) marks the Menopause transition as a several-year window. It begins with early perimenopause of variable length signaled by fluctuating follicle stimulating hormone (FSH) levels as declining estrogens from the ovaries fail to produce a negative feedback to the brain. A late perimenopause of one to three years is marked by consistently rising FSH levels as estrogen levels fall further, followed by early menopause which lasts for two to six years during which FSH levels stabilize at a high level into late menopause. But what has this to do with the many symptoms that women experience in this chapter of their lives? For those answers, we must examine the critical relationship that exists between estrogen and inflammation.

In the reproductive years, estradiol, 95% of which is produced by the ovaries, functions as the most powerful estrogen. It was always respected for its role in pregnancy and menstrual cycling. Yet, more recently, scientists have shown that during those years estradiol also serves to suppress the response to critical inflammatory proteins such as interleukin 1 (IL-1), interleukin 6 (IL-6) and tumor necrosis factor alpha (TNF a), which are normally generated by monocytes, macrophages, neutrophils, and other cell populations. These inflammatory proteins, when expressed, are capable of stimulating over 60 other inflammatory proteins that we now recognize attack brain, bone, heart, skin, and blood vessels. The appearance of these inflammatory proteins parallels the fluctuating and then rapidly declining estrogen levels seen in late perimenopause.

Women may recognize this period of their lives only by the onset of irregular menstrual periods. Yet it is during this window of time that estrogen levels fluctuate and even may increase briefly before beginning to decline permanently. It is also a time when some women for the first time begin to experience transient hot flashes, mood disorders, vaginal dryness, or sleep disorders.

From clinical studies, scientists also have shown that during the three to five years leading up to the last menstrual period, visceral fat that surrounds our abdominal organs and coats our blood vessels increases to a greater degree than does subcutaneous fat. These specialized fat cells act as tiny factories to produce a wide range of inflammatory proteins. These changes are accompanied by a rise in blood lipid levels and increases in blood vessel wall thickness. These cardiovascular events, while perhaps not generating the emotional reaction of many of the other perimenopausal symptoms, signal the real risk in menopause, that of a cardiovascular event and even stroke.

As scientists continue to clarify the biology of the menopause transition, they will offer clinicians and their patient's education and novel approaches to accommodate this most natural time in life.

THE STORY OF ESTROGEN: NOT JUST YOUR MOTHER'S HORMONE

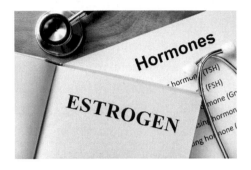

The story of the history of estrogen illustrates the historical progression of medical knowledge, from laboratory and clinical observation, through basic and clinical experimentation, to current successful medical management, an interesting marriage of empiricism and technology.

Our bodies efficiently make our natural hormones. Cholesterol from our diet is converted into a family of progesterones, which then become our androgens, such as testosterone, androstenedione, and dehydroepiandrosterone (DHEA). Androgens are important since they are the substrate for all of the estrogens in our body. The ovaries alone convert testosterone to estradiol (E2), the most powerful of the estrogens. Fat cells can convert androstenedione to other weaker estrogens, including estrone (E1), only 40% as active as estradiol, and estriol (E3), only 10% as active as estradiol. Since menopausal symptoms seem to arise with falling estrogen levels, estrogen has been sought as treatment of these symptoms.

How did estrogen come to dominate the discussion of menopause? In the late 1800s, knowledge of hormones was nonexistent, and medical decision-making was based solely on empirical observation. As a prelude to the discovery of other hormones, in the mid-1850s, Claude Bernard demonstrated that glands had internal secretions that could influence other organs. In 1897, ovarian extract was found to be effective for the treatment of menopausal hot flushing. Then, in 1906, secretions from the ovaries were shown to produce estrus (cyclic sexual activity in non-human females) and the term "estrogen" was born, derived from the Greek oistros (mad desire) and gennan (to produce). Yet, it was not until 1929 that estrogen as a hormone was isolated.

The first commercial preparation of estrogen began as an estrogen complex extracted from placentas called Emmenin, which was used to treat dysmenorrhea. The pharmaceutical company Ayerst, McKennen, and Harrison, Ltd. then developed Emmenin as the first oral female sex hormone. In 1938, an article appeared describing a similar collection of substances from pregnant mare urine (PMU). That publication led to the commercial production of PMU in 1939, at which point it was renamed Premarin® (pregnant-mare-urine). Premarin® contained at least ten estrogens, the dominant ones being estrone (50% to 60%) and equilin (22.5% to 32.5%) with less than 5% estradiol. Premarin® became commercially available in the United States (U.S.) in 1942. By 1992, Premarin® was the number one prescribed drug in the U.S., with sales exceeding $1 billion in 1997.

This changed drastically in July of 2002, when the release of results from the Women's Health Initiative (WHI) abruptly altered women's attitudes toward hormone replacement therapy (HRT). A documented statistical increase in breast cancer and stroke by menopausal women taking PremPro® (Premarin® and Provera®) led to many women abruptly stopping HRT with a resulting significant drop in prescriptions. This also fueled the search for a safer delivery system for estrogen.

Today, all of the major estrogens except Premarin® are derived from plants or synthesized denovo and are bioidentical hormones, i.e., identical in structure and function to the body's own estrogens. Most of these can be delivered transdermally or intravaginally. Why is this an advantage? All oral estrogens undergo a first pass through the liver via the portal system before entering the general circulation. This leads to a rise in inflammatory and procoagulant markers with a resultant increased risk of venous thrombosis. Transdermal estrogen significantly reduces these risks by entering the bloodstream directly, bypassing the liver. Progesterone, which is part of HRT given to decrease uterine cancer risk with estrogen alone, can be given intravaginally, transdermally, or perhaps via intrauterine device. It turns out that women without a uterus in the WHI, who therefore did not need the progesterone component of HRT, did not have a greater risk of cardiovascular accident (CVA) or myocardial infarction (MI). However, this was greatly downplayed at the time of the released data in 2002.

Improvements in the delivery and understanding of estrogen's role in

6

perimenopausal and postmenopausal women, including risks and benefits, have led to a better quality of life for women as their lifespan continues to increase. With further research and clinical study, this should only continue to improve.

WAS THE WOMEN'S HEALTH INITIATIVE GOOD OR BAD FOR WOMEN'S HEALTH?

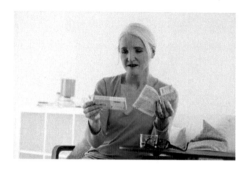

Most women are familiar with the Women's Health Initiative (WHI), the largest randomized controlled trial to date, which was sponsored by the National Institute of Health (NIH) to evaluate the role of hormone therapy in menopause to protect cardiovascular and bone health. Begun in 1991 as a proposed 15-year study, women in menopause with a uterus were randomized to take orally either a placebo or PremPro®, a combination of Premarin®, a conjugated equine estrogen (CEE) and medroxyprogesterone, a synthetic version of progesterone. Women with a hysterectomy were given either CEE alone or placebo. In part, this $725 million study was intended to resolve the controversy over whether menopause should be embraced as a natural transition in life, a position taken by the feminist movement at the time, or, as proposed by such books as *Feminine Forever* (Pocket Books, NY, 1968), that menopause was a hormone deficiency totally preventable with hormone therapy.

In 2002, the entire study was abruptly stopped due to a statistical increase in breast cancer and stroke and no apparent benefit for reducing cardiovascular risk. This bold action by the NIH prompted the New York Times article entitled, "Hormone Replacement Study: A Shock to the Medical System." As one physician later wrote, "I may have taken my last pill this morning." By 2003, there was a precipitous reduction in hormone prescriptions, ushering in a decade of menopausal women without hormone support. But was the WHI study done correctly?

The purpose of hormone replacement in menopause is to compensate for the lack of estrogen, primarily estradiol, of which 95% is produced by the ovaries during the reproductive years. The role of a progestin is to duplicate progesterone, produced cyclically by the premenopausal ovaries, whose sole purpose is to prevent overstimulation of the uterine lining by estradiol.

Three aspects of the WHI deserve closer scrutiny: the age of the women in the study, the choice of the hormones used, and the significance of the statistical risk.

With an average age of 63 years, many of these women participating in the study may already have had vascular damage from age-related changes, thus increasing their risks for cardiovascular events. The average age of menopause in the United States is 51 years.

In the WHI, Premarin®, derived from the urine of pregnant mares (Pre-mar-in) contains ten different estrogens but almost no estradiol, the most powerful of the body's estrogens. Taken as an estrogen pill, it is absorbed in the intestine, with a "first pass" through the liver, increasing production of many clotting factors. This explains the increased incidence of stroke in both arms of the study. Conversely, transdermal estrogen does not stimulate these clotting factors. Medroxyprogesterone was used as the progestin. This is a synthetic chemical version of progesterone. Women on PremPro® did show a statistical increase in breast cancer. Yet, those women with a hysterectomy, and therefore taking Premarin® only, showed a reduction in breast cancer mortality. Was it the progestin? Recent data suggests that medroxyprogesterone in breast tissue may alter hormone receptors adjacent to the estrogen receptors, thus increasing the risks of estrogen-stimulated cancers.

Applying statistical risk to clinical risk also is a challenge. In the WHI, out of 10,000 person-years, there were seven more cardiac events, eight more strokes, eight more pulmonary emboli, and eight more breast cancers. The WHI frightened women (a negative), but it laid the groundwork for improved menopausal care (a positive). Today, there is a growing sense that if women are started on hormone replacement in their late 40s or early 50s and are administered pure estradiol by a patch or cream and pure progesterone, that the original hypotheses of the WHI might have been better served.

MENOPAUSE, METABOLISM, AND VISCERAL FAT ACCUMULATION

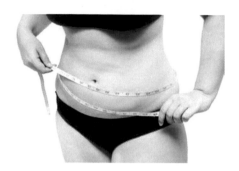

Our bodies, anthropologically, function solely to reproduce in order to preserve our species. But reproduction requires adequate metabolic energy. Witness the increase in body fat as one enters puberty or the negative effect on fertility for patients with anorexia nervosa, for those engaging in strenuous exercise, or those subjected to famine and starvation. Yet, as our ability to reproduce ceases at the other end of the age spectrum, we experience a reduction in metabolism, redistribution of fat to our abdominal area and, thus, the cardiovascular and diabetic risks of metabolic syndrome. The key to these interactions resides in our hypothalamus where reproduction and metabolism are controlled.

Reproduction is initiated by three small groups of neurons in our hypothalamus called the KNDy neurons (kisspeptin, neurokinin B, and dynorphin) pronounced "candy." In the adolescent child, as puberty approaches, suppressor genes that have kept these neurons quiet since birth lose their inhibitory effect. These KNDy neurons, with direct connections to our gonadotrophin-releasing hormone (GnRH) neurons, stimulate the release of gonadotrophin-releasing hormone (GnRH). GnRH, in turn, activates the pituitary to produce pulsatile luteinizing hormone (LH) and follicle-stimulating hormone (FSH), both of which stimulate the ovaries to begin to produce cyclic estrogen and progesterone, and the reproductive cycle begins.

These KNDy neurons, however, also play an important role in regulating metabolism by responding to feedback from peripheral hormones that are responsible for appetite and nutritional absorption. While more complex than stated here, in brief, leptin released from our white fat and insulin from our pancreas decrease our appetite and tell us to eat less. In contrast, ghrelin, from our gut, increases our appetite, usually causing us to eat more.

Evidence that our metabolism and reproductive function interact is demonstrated by the fact that caloric restriction leading to ghrelin secretion reduces pulsatile GnRH release from the gonadotrophin-releasing neurons, thereby impairing ovulation. Although metabolism and reproduction must work collaboratively, reproductive processes do not respond directly to metabolic cues. For example, GnRH neurons have no leptin or ghrelin receptors, and KNDy neurons have no ghrelin receptors. The higher order control of metabolism to support reproduction is believed to reside at the arcuate nucleus in the hypothalamus, which has access to circulating molecules outside the blood-brain barrier. It also has receptors for leptin, insulin, and ghrelin, and contains regulators of the KNDy and GnRH neurons.

Connecting the dots, however, has left us with one question: "Why does visceral fat form in the months or years leading into menopause?"

The initiating factor may be fluctuation and then loss of ovarian estradiol with its anti-inflammatory properties in the menopause transition, thus altering the immune characteristics of our intestinal bacteria and their control over nutritional absorption. Falling estradiol levels also produce alterations in KNDy neurons (now believed to be the origin of hot flashes) and could facilitate changes in how we metabolize our food. Evidence supporting this theory is found in breast cancer patients treated with aromatase inhibitors who have lowered estrogen levels and both an increasing incidence of hot flashes and increasing abdominal obesity. A contrasting theory, supported by animal and clinical studies, indicates an association between higher androgen levels and visceral fat accumulation. Perhaps both low estrogen and relatively elevated androgen levels contribute to the development of metabolic syndrome phenotype in genetically predisposed perimenopausal women. Other hormones, like thyroid hormone and cortisol, obviously have some role in this process as well.

Visceral fat cells, although only a small component of our overall body fat, accumulate non-esterified free fatty acids faster than subcutaneous fat cells. These visceral fat cells deliver free fatty acids (FFA) via the portal vein directly to our liver, thus contributing a higher proportion of overall hepatic FFA in individuals with greater visceral fat. The results are an increase in very low density lipoproteins (VLDL) and insulin resistance, hallmarks of type 2 diabetes and increased cardiovascular risk.

The biologies of reproduction and of metabolism, once thought of as silos, now seem more integrated. This observation raises new possibilities for novel treatments to prevent metabolic syndrome.

METABOLIC SYNDROME AND
THE ROLE OF ESTROGEN

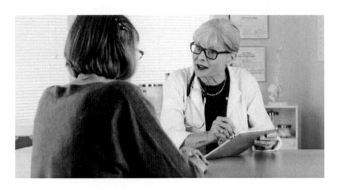

Metabolic syndrome represents a cluster of adverse biologic events characterized by alterations in lipids, elevated blood sugar, and increased cardiovascular risk. According to the National Cholesterol Education Program's Adult Treatment Panel 111 Report, metabolic syndrome may be diagnosed when three of the following criteria are present: waist circumference greater than 88 cm, HDL-C less than 50 mg/dL, triglycerides greater than 150 mg/dL, blood pressure above 130/85 mmHg, or fasting blood sugar over 110 mg/dL. The greatest health risk of metabolic syndrome is cardiovascular disease, but this risk also is age related. Sixty percent of postmenopausal women are affected by metabolic syndrome, whereas only 22% of the general population meet these criteria. These differences in prevalence underscore the dramatic physiologic changes that occur as a woman enters menopause.

Menopause is defined as one year without menses. The menopause transition now is formally defined as the three-to-five-year period leading up to this new stage of life. This transition often is recognized by women with the onset of irregular menses and vasomotor symptoms. Often, it is characterized by increased fat depositions, especially in the intra-abdominal area (visceral fat) with little change in muscle mass. Visceral fat cells with direct access to portal blood entering the liver are a significant source of many of the inflammatory proteins felt to be responsible for cardiovascular heart disease. The appearance of these inflammatory proteins results from fluctuations and then the natural decline of ovarian estradiol, a hormone that in the pre-menopause provides anti-inflammatory protection.

Visceral obesity also correlates closely with an increase in insulin resistance leading to elevated insulin levels, abnormal glucose metabolism, and a reduction in fat breakdown. Insulin, acting through its receptors to stimulate insulin-like growth factor-2 (IGF2), is critical for normal glucose metabolism. It transports glucose from the blood into the cells and allows fat to be broken down. Yet, insulin receptors are under hormonal control since estradiol improves insulin sensitivity and glucose metabolism while reducing body fat. Obesity, coupled with insulin resistance, results in over expression of insulin receptors, lower than normal levels of IGF-2, and production of a second growth factor, insulin-like growth factor -1 (IGF-1), which causes a pathologic process that destabilizes glucose metabolism in insulin-sensitive tissue.

Visceral fat also has a direct effect to increase appetite and reduce energy expenditure. Premenopausal estradiol maintains a balance of intestinal peptides that signal the brain when a person has eaten enough. In these women, appetite is controlled by increased adiponectin and ghrelin and decreased resistin and leptin. Yet, in obese women with metabolic syndrome and insulin resistance, adiponectin (important for cardiovascular protection) is decreased, and leptin and resistin are increased. How do we know estradiol is involved? Transdermal estradiol supplementation in these women reverses these changes. Moreover, in clinical studies, energy expenditure in obese women with metabolic syndrome is reduced but improves once transdermal estradiol supplementation is instituted.

It is not surprising that obesity, especially in the menopause transition, appears to be the primary clinical target for reducing the risk from the metabolic syndrome. Daily exercise and diet management to reduce fat, especially visceral fat, is central to this effort. Moreover, hormone supplementation with transdermal estradiol capitalizes on the effect of estradiol to increase insulin sensitivity, reduce abdominal fat, and rebalance intestinal satiety peptides.

WHAT DO WE KNOW ABOUT HOT FLASHES IN MENOPAUSE?

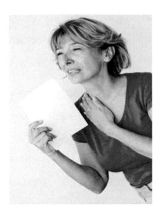

It is 3 am, and while in bed, you are awakened by a sudden burst of heat in your face, neck, and arms that forces you, now drenched in sweat, to throw off the covers, only then to chill. With up to 75% of women experiencing this phenomenon during the menopause transition and 10% for a lifetime, what do we know about the biology of hot flashes?

Hot flashes are initiated by enhanced sympathetic activity within the brain in association with reduced ovarian estrogen production. Yet, the occurrence of hot flashes correlates poorly with measured levels of plasma, urinary or vaginal estrogen. Hot flashes, however, are linked to elevated baseline plasma levels of norepinephrine metabolites in symptomatic women, which increase further during a hot flash. Estrogen's actions in the brain during ovulation to reduce the response of sympathetic receptors may explain why, during estrogen withdrawal, enhanced sympathetic activity occurs. But how does this explain the clinical picture of hot flashes?

Scientists have found that, during the reproductive years, a woman can adjust to a change in her environment of about 0.4 degrees C without stimulating the hypothalamus, the thermoregulatory part of her brain. Entering a warm room, smoking a cigarette, or having spicy food; these events do not seem to stimulate a central sympathetic response. This is referred to as the "thermoneutral zone." Yet, in the menopausal years, coincidental with a drop in estrogen levels, the thermoneutral zone disappears. This change has been reproduced in the animal model where administering norepinephrine into the blood stream also narrows the thermoneutral zone. Any small rise in temperature then triggers the hypothalamus into action with the goal to lower the body's temperature. As a result, one's heart rate increases to direct capillary blood flow to the skin and moisture is released through the sweat glands, both intended to reduce one's body temperature. Then a brief drop in body temperature occurs, the chill factor.

Treatments using cognitive behavioral therapy, or mind-body interventions such as yoga, hypnosis, or acupuncture, effectively reduce one's response to hot flashes but have little or no effect on frequency. Nonetheless, these approaches have been shown to improve one's response to stress, sleep disorders, and depression. Moreover, dietary modification and weight loss have been shown to reduce vasomotor symptoms.

Estrogen is the gold standard medication for treating hot flashes, usually reducing their incidence and severity. The effectiveness of other treatments must be judged against their placebo effect, the lessening of symptoms based on the woman's expectation that the treatment will work. For those who cannot take systemic estrogens, treatment with clonidine; the Selective Serotonin Reuptake inhibitors (SSRIs) fluoxetine, paroxetine, or sertraline; or the anticonvulsant gabapentin, have all been reported to reduce hot flashes from 20% to 50% of women tested.

DOCTOR, WHY DOES IT HURT DOWN THERE?

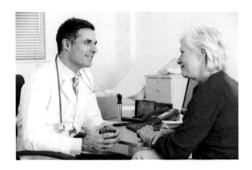

Over 60% of women in menopause complain, often silently, of vaginal dryness and pain during intercourse. As a consequence, they may seek to avoid that level of intimacy, a behavior that can impact negatively on their relationships and, for some, may lead to loneliness and depression. Why?

During the reproductive years, estradiol, produced by the ovaries, is important for health of the vagina, vulva, and lower bladder. Estradiol stimulates nitric oxide, a dilator of blood vessels, to deliver blood with its high water content to the pelvis. This moisture is drawn into the tissues because of the differing concentrations of sodium, potassium, and chloride between blood and vaginal secretions. These ions are important for regulating vaginal lubrication. Estradiol also stimulates the growth of lactobacillis, healthy vaginal bacteria that metabolize glycogen anaerobically to lactic acid in order to maintain the acidity of the vagina at 4 +/- .05, a pH that is hostile to many sexually transmitted infections. Deeper within the tissues, estradiol protects collagen to maintain support and integrity of the vagina, vulva, and bladder.

During menopause, vaginal tissues become dry and shrink. Why? Estradiol's decline results in a reversal of its tissue-protecting effects. Blood vessels decrease in number and size, thus, reducing tissue moisture. Lactobacillis that formerly maintained acidity of the vagina disappear, leading to more alkaline vaginal secretions (normal postmenopausal vaginal pH is 6 to 7.5) and a greater risk of infections. Even the bladder becomes more susceptible to urinary tract infections (UTI). But what makes the vaginal area so vulnerable to these infections? That question takes us to the heart of the problem.

Declining levels of ovarian estradiol lead to chronic inflammation in these tissues, as other cells begin to produce inflammatory proteins that had been chronically suppressed by higher levels of estrogens during the reproductive years. It is the emergence of inflammation in the vaginal area that promotes the repeating infections that women experience. It also explains the pain on intercourse, as vaginal manipulation occurs in the setting of these inflamed tissues.

Systemic hormone replacement may reduce vaginal dryness, but it is not for everyone. Local hormonal therapy in the form of estradiol cream applied to the vagina in small amounts reverses many of these inflammatory-induced effects. However, some women, especially breast cancer survivors, usually are told not to use vaginal estrogen cream due to their risk of increased estrogen blood levels above the normal menopausal range. Yet, due to the estrogen-blocking drugs that many breast cancer survivors take, the problems of vaginal dryness are greater than those of normal menopausal women. Current studies now indicate that androgen creams made of testosterone or dehydroepiandrosterone (DHEA) may offer relief without increasing estrogen blood levels.

Vaginal dryness affects the majority of menopausal women. Fortunately, systemic hormone therapy and local therapies such as estrogen and androgen creams, moisturizers, lubricants, and pH balancers now are available to help.

WHY IS MENOPAUSE MANAGEMENT NOT BETTER UNDERSTOOD BY OB/GYN CARE PROVIDERS?

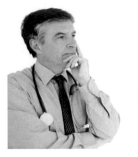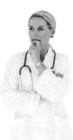

Today, menopause management as a finite field of medicine is a product of many laboratory and clinical studies targeted at understanding the biology of menopause and the impact of hormonal and non-hormonal treatments. Why, then, do women in the menopausal transition or in menopause itself often confront a medical community that is either not aware of or is even indifferent to the challenges they face?

The concept of menopause is not new. Symptoms of menopause in midlife were observed in women as far back as the time of Aristotle. By 1921, the term "menopause" gave this time of life a name. However, women's psychosocial issues were slow to gain recognition, perhaps because gynecologic care was provided by mostly male physicians in an era of paternalistic medicine. Evidence the debate in the 1970s as to whether premenstrual dysphoria actually existed. The concept that symptoms of menopause might begin months or years before that one year without a menstrual period (officially called menopause) or that the symptoms for some women might last well into their 70s was not discussed.

In 1968, Robert Wilson, a gynecologist in New York City, published *Feminine Forever* advocating that menopause was a discrete time of life and was treatable. In his own words, "The often-severe suffering of my menopausal patients made me regard menopause as a serious medical condition endangering the health and happiness of any woman...In the vast majority of cases the distressing bodily changes following menopause are reversible through estrogen treatment." Unfortunately, by portraying menopause as a "disease to be treated," he inflamed the feminist movement, which at that time was advocating menopause as a natural transition in life to be tolerated and even embraced.

It was out of that debate that in 1992 the Women's Health Initiative was funded by the National Institutes of Health (NIH) to study hormone replacement and its potential preventive actions. Those results and subsequent study-analyses, fueled by the pharmaceutical industry, spawned a wide range of treatments for menopause. Around that same time, in 1989, the North American Menopause Society was formed, bringing together scientists and physicians in OB/GYN and general medicine with a goal to "promote the health and quality of life of all women during midlife and beyond through an understanding of menopause and healthy aging."

Even with these efforts, why do women patients still ask, "Why is menopause not better understood by care providers?" Here are four possible answers. 1. Formal training in OB/GYN is usually clinic based, involving younger patients with a focus on obstetrics, contraception, and sexually transmitted infections. 2. The practice of OB/GYN demands that the practitioner acquires a wide range of surgical skills for managing obstetric care and gynecologic surgery. Menopause management is not dominated by the requirement of manual surgical skills. 3. Menopause management in the office is time-intensive in an era when insurance reimbursement rewards procedures and shorter visits with higher numbers of patients seen. 4. Menopause management requires more individualization of education and treatment, which is, by itself, a higher level skill in medicine. This form of practice is more trial and error than much of medicine and requires patience by clinician and patient, an emotion which is often in short supply in our world of short attention spans.

Is there a brighter future for menopause care? Efforts are underway to improve research, therapeutics, and gynecologic care to address the needs of educated menopausal women. As more women care providers age and become more interested in menopause medicine, patients will benefit. In addition, women themselves will bring about change as they become better educated about menopause management. Menopause is a time of life, NOT a disease.

INTIMACY AND THE BREAST CANCER SURVIVOR

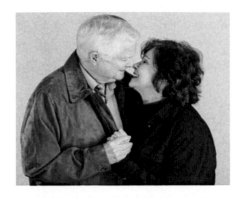

Early detection and directed treatments have led to improved outcomes for women with breast cancer. Nonetheless, the gynecologic impact of these treatments is significant. In one study, 42% of breast cancer survivors experienced vaginal dryness, 38% reported that intercourse was painful, and 64% felt loss of libido. For many women, these changes affect her relationship with her partner directly, thereby increasing her risk of depression. Furthermore, medical treatment for depression can accelerate loss of sexual interest and further endanger the relationship. In one series, when 610 breast cancer survivors with normal sexual activity were given antidepressants, 57% experienced loss of libido.

For menopausal women without breast cancer, systemic or vaginal estrogens have been the treatment of choice for vaginal dryness and pain during intercourse. The dilemma facing the breast cancer survivor is that in vitro, animal, and human clinical studies document that long-term estrogen exposure is linked to the development, progression, and recurrence of breast cancer. In fact, aromatase inhibitors and tamoxifen, which block estrogen, often are used prophylactically for five to ten years after immediate breast cancer treatment. Consistent with this anti-estrogen approach, the medical community has been forced to adopt a "no hormone for you" stance for breast cancer survivors.

Efforts to evaluate the role of vaginal estrogen for breast cancer survivors have produced mixed results, but at least one small study has reported that vaginal estrogen in certain women can elevate circulating blood estrogen levels above that observed normally in menopause. Are there other approaches? Vaginal testosterone and DHEA creams have been tested clinically, and neither increases the circulating levels of estrogen above menopausal levels. The biologic benefits draw from the fact that the androgens applied to the vagina are not acting through an androgen receptor but most likely are being converted to estrogens at the local tissue level. Nonetheless, monitoring estrogen blood levels is a critical part of this management. Neither, however, is FDA approved for this purpose currently.

Most patients using either of these androgen creams experience less vaginal dryness, a lower vaginal pH, and increased moisture. Water-based gels are available if the vehicle used in the compounded androgen cream or gel generates local irritation. Many of these women again find intercourse less uncomfortable.

Survivors of breast cancer treatment have a very challenging journey made more complicated by the fact that many of these treatments have an impact on the couple's relationship. This new information about the use of androgens for treating vaginal dryness and pain on intercourse for breast cancer survivors does not address all of the symptoms of treatment-induced menopause, but it provides some local solutions to vaginal dryness and pain.

ESTROGEN AND BREAST CANCER:
A LOVE-HATE RELATIONSHIP

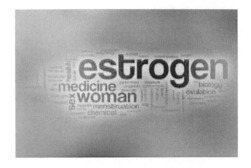

What do the dates 1896 and 1935 have to do with breast cancer? They mark critical moments in clarifying the complex relationship between estrogen and breast cancer. Breast cancer is the second leading cause of cancer mortality in the United States and Canada. Understanding its relationship to estrogen is critical for attributing cause and planning future therapies.

In 1896, it was observed that breast cancer regressed if women had both ovaries removed (surgical menopause) or progressed into natural menopause, even though estrogen had not yet been discovered as a hormone. In 1916, this relationship was demonstrated in the animal model, and in 1923 estrogen was identified and named.

Clinical studies reinforced the concept that length of estrogen exposure affected breast cancer risk. Risk factors include women with early onset menses or late menopause, women who do not have children or who have had children later in life, women who do not breastfeed, obese women, and those who abuse alcohol. The estrogen-induced biologic pathway leading to breast cancer has been shown to involve estrogen-related gene mutations and generation of reactive oxygen species.

At odds with this process is the fact that in The Women's Health Initiative (WHI) report of 2002, women with a hysterectomy who were given only conjugated estrogen (Premarin®) and not the combination of Premarin® and the synthetic progestin, medroxyprogesterone acetate (as PremPro®), showed a reduction in breast cancer incidence and mortality compared to controls. It appears that under certain circumstances, estrogen protects against breast cancer. How could this be?

Haddo, a British microbiologist, first demonstrated in his laboratory that under certain circumstances some synthetic estrogens, one being diethylstilbestrol (DES), can retard growth of breast cancer cells and later confirmed this finding in a clinical trial. By the 1960s, DES in high doses was being used to treat breast cancer, producing a reduction in breast cancer cells in one-third of women. However, for breast cancer survivors at least five years into menopause and therefore deprived of estrogen for an extended period, estrogen's action to kill breast cancer cells was more striking than that for younger women.

The science of breast cancer is changing continuously. Evidence is accruing that while breast cancer in most cases does involve a lifetime of estrogen exposure, if those breast cancer cells are deprived of estrogen for an extended period, they change, and estrogen then becomes a "lethal bullet." This concept appears radical but in time may provide new approaches to the treatment of breast cancer.

ARE ALL BREAST CANCERS THE SAME?
A Paradox – Estrogen's Relationship to Breast Cancer

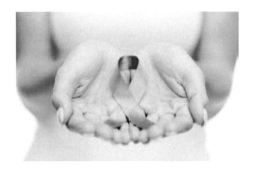

Most women are aware of a link between estrogen and breast cancer. Yet, there are different types of breast cancer i.e., ductal, lobular, inflammatory, with various receptor characteristics that guide treatment. Approximately 75% of breast cancer is estrogen receptor (ER) positive. However, there are conditions in which estrogen both fuels and at other times kills ER-positive breast cancer cells. One type of breast cancer does not even recognize estrogen at all. In 2011, there were 230,480 new cases of breast cancer and 57,650 cases of breast carcinoma in situ while 29,520 women were predicted to die of this disease. Understanding the types of breast cancer offers promise for improved surveillance, prevention and more effective treatments.

Observers noted as early as 1896 that the ovaries were related to breast cancer since some women with breast cancer improved after their ovaries were removed. Yet, it was not until 1923 that estrogen as a hormone was discovered. While estrogen can stimulate growth of certain breast cancer cells, if these cells are deprived of hormones for five years by anti-estrogen medication, they are made vulnerable to being killed by estrogen through cell apoptosis. This may explain the cancer-killing effect of diethylstilbesterol (DES) in the 1960s when one third of women with breast cancer given the drug improved.

Duration of exposure to estrogen over a woman's lifetime relates to the risk for developing estrogen-receptor positive breast cancer. This form of breast cancer is more common in women with early onset menses, late onset menopause, and nulliparity or having children later in life. All of these situations involve prolonged menstrual cycling and estrogen exposure. Other risk factors are lack of breastfeeding, alcohol consumption (which increases estrogen production) and obesity, since adipose cells produce estrogen. Additional factors are smoking, family history, and genetic status.

The association of ER-positive breast cancer to lifelong estrogen exposure helps explain why such women are usually older at cancer onset. In the Women's Health Initiative (WHI), the average age of participants was 63. Estrogen in the form of Premarin plus the synthetic progestin, medroxyprogesterone (PremPro), given to women who still had their uterus, increased overall breast cancer risk. Yet, in women without a uterus, estrogen replacement therapy alone (ERT) decreased the overall breast cancer risk. Whether the synthetic progestin in the first group contributed to the increase in breast cancer remains unclear. In the second group, estrogen was not started until nearly 10 years after menopause, so a period of estrogen deprivation preceding the estrogen-only exposure may have induced apoptosis of nascent cancer cells.

Certain other breast cancers do not express the common hormone receptor genes for estrogen, progesterone or the newer marker, human epidermal growth factor (HER2). Called triple-negative breast cancer (TNBC), this cancer, first reported in 2005, often occurs in younger women, even during their reproductive years, and appears to be more aggressive. In one study, 33.8% of women under 40 with breast cancer were TNBC, while only 21.5% were ER positive. Yet, for all types of breast cancer, 23.9% of women were younger, while 76.1% were older.

Understanding the characteristics of these breast cancers challenges current protocols for surveillance and management. Controversy exists as to when to begin providing mammography to women. Administering estrogen after five years of anti-estrogen treatment may provide additional protection for ER-positive breast cancer survivors. In fact, ongoing studies of anti-estrogen treatment alternating with ERT or "drug holidays" may answer some of these questions. Medical science is built on questions leading to answers that ask more questions. Progress in breast cancer research exemplifies this process.

BRCA GENES: PROTECTOR FROM OR CAUSE OF BREAST CANCER?

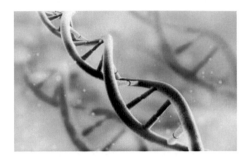

Many women have heard of the term "BRCA" standing for Breast Cancer Associated genes and their association with inherited breast cancers. Perhaps not as well-known is the fact that the BRCA genes normally play an important role in protecting our bodies as they age. It is only when mutations of these BRCA genes occur that the risk for developing cancer increases, because the mutations inactivate their protective effects.

Throughout our lifetime, our body continually is engaged in renewing itself. Every minute, somewhere in our body our aging cells pass on their "personality" by creating "daughter cells" that will replace them in location and function. Old cardiac cells produce identical but younger heart cells. Old muscle cells generate newer muscle cells and so on. These amazing events occur through a process called deoxyribonucleic acid (DNA) replication.

The genetic makeup for each cell in our body is contained in a double-stranded DNA molecule. Each time a cell divides, the two resulting daughter cells each receive the same genetic information that was contained in the DNA of the parent cell, but it is the organization of the DNA that gives it its genomic identity. The two strands of the DNA, which provide the backbone of the molecule, are connected by bonding of strand components called nucleotides, arranged like steps on a ladder. The nucleotides, adenine (A) and thymine (T), always pair with one another, as do the nucleotides, cytosine (C) and guanine (G). The specific arrangement of these pairs of nucleotides along the double-stranded DNA, like a computer code, produces the unique genetic fingerprint of that cell.

The process by which daughter cells are provided the identical genetic makeup of the parent cell begins as the two DNA strands in the parent cell are separated, much as a zipper is unzipped, leaving each strand with its own complement of half paired nucleotides, bearing all necessary information to make a new cell. While each strand is open, free-floating nucleotides present in the cellular environment that normally pair with those specific nucleotides are secured, thus reestablishing the paired relationship. Finally, enzymes reassemble the new strands into a double-coiled arrangement in each of the daughter cells. Since each time a cell divides it has to copy and transmit the exact sequence of more than three billion nucleotides to its daughter cells, it is easy to understand the risks of transmitting mistakes to the next generation of cells.

It is in the governing of this process that BRCA genes normally play an important role. DNA replication occurs in an orderly fashion dictated by progression through a cell cycle made up of five steps designated G0 (resting), G1 (first gap), S (synthesis), G2 (second gap), and M (mitosis) phases. Each phase is separated by a checkpoint in which transition from one step to the next mandates that all requirements at that checkpoint are satisfied. If at any checkpoint problems are encountered, the cell cycle is stopped until repairs are made. The undamaged BRCA genes oversee this repair process.

There are five known repair pathways which can be activated when ultraviolet light, cosmic or isotopic irradiation, environmental pollution, cigarette smoking, or other insults damage our DNA. Two important mechanisms are homologous recombination repair (HRR) and non-homologous enjoining (NHEJ). BRCA genes participate in both, specializing in the rejoining of double-stranded DNA that has been cut clean through, leaving the chromosome in two pieces. Non-homologous enjoining ligates DNA damaged ends in G1 phase by removing or adding bases to the broken ends. Homologous recombination repair only functions at the checkpoint between S and G2. Rejoining broken chromosomal DNA suppresses the uncontrolled replication of breast cells leading to a malignant tumor.

Inherited mutations of the BRCA1 and BRCA2 genes, identified in 1990 and 1995 respectively, inactivate the repair capacity of the genes, removing this protective shield. Significantly, since inherited BRCA mutations come from the germ line that is the source of all cells in the body, they greatly increase cancer risk. In the case of breast cells, all have the mutation, and so all are impaired in DNA strand joining.

The clinical implications have been recognized only recently. Today, in the general population, there is a 12% lifetime risk for breast cancer, yet by age 70 there is a 55% to 65% risk of breast cancer if one carries a BRCA1 mutation and a 45% risk with a BRCA2 mutation. Lifetime risk for ovarian cancer in the general population is 1.3%, but 39% of women with the BRCA1 mutations and 11% to 17% with the BRCA2 mutations will develop ovarian cancer by age 70.

How has this information helped women? Advances in cancer management have resulted from risk identity, improved surveillance, and targeted treatments. Genetic research and engineering, as well as expanding our knowledge of the health and risks to our DNA, focus on all three areas of science.

CAN SOME CANCER PATIENTS TAKE HORMONE REPLACEMENT THERAPY?

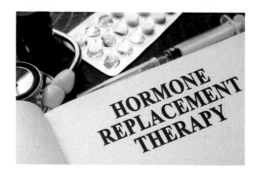

When someone receives the diagnosis of cancer, life changes forever. Just one minute before, that individual and her family led normal lives. Never more. They suddenly are flooded with questions. "What does this mean? What can be done? Do I need a second opinion? Do I need surgery, chemotherapy, radiation therapy, and/or immunotherapy? Am I going to die? And again, what did you just say?"

Our fear of cancer drives much of our preventive health care. Mammograms, Pap smears, annual examinations, colonoscopies, all are targeted at ruling out cancer. As affirmation of these efforts, however, the National Cancer Institute reports that the number of people living after a cancer diagnosis was almost 14.5 million in 2014 and is expected to rise to almost 19 million by 2024. How we follow these people and improve their quality of life is a work in progress.

For many women, the aftermath of several treatments for cancer involves the loss of reproductive capabilities and cessation of hormone production. Because of radiation, chemotherapy, and/or surgery to remove the uterus and ovaries, many women find themselves thrust into menopause. With the loss of ovarian estradiol, these women are likely to experience menopausal symptoms including hot flashes, mood swings, sleep disorders, bone loss, and vaginal atrophy. For some, the symptoms may be so acute as to lead them to consider whether the benefits of hormone replacement therapy (HRT) are more desirable than the possibility that hormone supplementation may enhance the risks of cancer recurrence or the occurrence of a new cancer.

Absent cancer, those same women at some stage of their lives may benefit from hormone replacement therapy. A common response from many care providers is, "No hormones for you, because of your cancer." That common response is not exactly true as newer research demonstrates. Nonetheless, accepting conclusions of most cancer studies must be tempered by whether the hormones used were estrogen replacement therapy (ERT) only (women with hysterectomy) or estrogen plus progesterone (HRT), as well as differences in age of study participants, type and degree of cancer stage, length of observation, confounding health issues, and changing treatments over time. Still, a trend seems to be developing that underscores possible differences in a variety of cancers for women who receive estrogen alone versus those who are given estrogen and progesterone.

Breast cancer is the most common cancer in women of all races. In the 1940s and 1950s, women with advanced or metastatic breast cancer were treated with high-dose estrogen (diethylstilbestrol-DES) with one-third of women responding favorably. Many years later, while women from the Women's Health Initiative (WHI) given HRT with Premarin® and medroxyprogesterone (PremPro®) showed a small increase in breast cancer over non-treated women, those with a hysterectomy receiving estrogen replacement therapy (ERT) only (Premarin®) showed a reduced incidence of breast cancer. Young women who carry BRCA mutations who elect to remove their fallopian tubes and ovaries prophylactically after childbearing and who choose to take ERT have not been found to have an increased risk in breast cancer in small studies.

Lung cancer is the second most frequent cancer among white and black women and third among Hispanic women. In a meta-analysis of 14 cohort studies, no increased risk was found for developing lung cancer if HRT (not defined) was used. When a prospective cohort of 36,588 women with lung cancer was studied, the combination of estrogen plus progesterone (HRT) increased the risk of incident lung cancer, but estrogen alone (ERT) produced no such association.

Colorectal cancer is the second most common cancer among Hispanic women and third among white and black women. From a cohort of 7,701 women who were initially free of cancer but were placed on estrogen only replacement therapy, ERT was associated with a reduced cancer risk when compared with non-users.

Endometrial cancer is the most treatable of women's cancers. Standard treatment consists of removal of the uterus and ovaries, along with a sampling of lymph nodes. In one study of 1,236 endometrial cancer survivors, of which 618 were placed on ERT versus those on placebo after surgery and followed for 35.7 months, the recurrence rate was very low, 3.1% in the placebo group and 0.6% in the ERT group.

Ovarian cancer recurrence risk with ERT was examined in the Adjuvant Hormone Therapy trial initiated in 1990. One hundred and fifty women were studied, with 75 using ERT and 75 as non-users. Estrogen replacement therapy users exhibited fewer recurrences, longer disease-free intervals, and improved survival.

Cervical cancer recurrences and HRT was studied in 120 survivors after surgery and/ or radiotherapy for stage 1 and 2 cancers. No significant increase in recurrences or survival was observed for HRT users (N=80) compared with non–users (N=40).

The safety of HRT versus ERT to treat menopausal symptoms in cancer survivors will never be absolute until our understanding of what causes cancer is complete. Why ERT only, as opposed to HRT, would seem to offer some protection against cancer of most types remains an enigma. One could postulate that the anti-inflammatory properties of estrogen reduce the incidence of mutation-derived cell change. Despite lacking a clear explanation, the emotional trauma of learning one has cancer should not, de facto, prevent a discussion of available studies of hormone therapy for menopausal symptoms. All a cancer survivor wants is to live a life of quality. Care providers should use that as a guide.

BREAST CANCER: TRAGEDY, FOLLOWED BY DISCOVERY, THEN PLAYED FORWARD

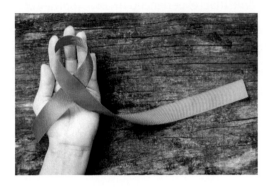

This short article, sent anonymously by a gynecologist to the periFACTS OB/GYN Academy, describes one man's journey to discovery.

I am a physician, a husband, a father, and a grandfather. Many years ago, at the age of 43, my former wife was diagnosed with triple-negative breast cancer and died at age 47. Our journey began the day before Valentine's Day when her mammogram was scheduled. I had ordered flowers to be delivered the next day. What should have been a perfect Valentine's Day instead was filled with phone calls to a surgeon and an oncologist regarding how to manage breast cancer.

While outsiders might have felt sympathy, sadness, even pity, could they really understand the significance of those next four years? The path my wife and I took can truly be appreciated only by those who have traveled it.

Of course, those four years tested me and my family, but no one more than my wife. A brilliant writer, she was reduced to confusing the oxygen tube for the music head set. She struggled to use phrases that she previously had written in elegant prose hundreds of times, all the while fighting to journal her inner thoughts, fears, and needs. Faced with the inevitable, her intent was to write cards to her family to be opened years later during birthdays, marriages, or births. Unbeknown to me at the time, she never succeeded in that task, and I searched for months, hoping unsuccessfully to find those cherished messages.

It was during the last three months of her life that I left medicine to become her complete care provider. Her mother and father, estranged for over 20 years by a vitriolic divorce, finally reunited at her bedside; no trauma or theatrics, only two parents saying goodbye to their daughter.

And it was during that time that I experienced my own journey of discovery, not knowing if I would have the strength or patience to take on this new role. Yet, when my wife was angry, I became her consoler. When she was sad, I was there to lift her up. When she finally passed peacefully, an outsider might mistakenly have imagined my sense of relief. That did not happen. During those last few months, so completely immersed in her care, I found my real purpose in life, my inner strength, and my ability to tolerate the intolerable. In the weeks following her passing, I felt stripped of my role, even as I had resumed my medical practice and, for any outsider, probably appeared to be engaged in life once more.

Today I am happily remarried with a full life. But one might ask if back then the journey my wife and I shared left me with a purpose? I am a better husband, father, and physician for having known her. I no longer feel awkward seeing patients and their families who are struggling with their own experiences. In fact, sitting and listening are often my best contributions to their plight. I cherish that gift.

Most breast cancer survivors want the life they had always hoped they would have. And they want to be respected as women despite the treatments they have endured. The gynecologist has the opportunity to provide a holistic approach to satisfy these wishes and to be part of the care team.

Signed: Anonymous

EXTENDED DISCUSSIONS

MAMMOGRAPHY AND BREAST CANCER SCREENING

Avice M. O'Connell, M.D., F.A.C.R.

INTRODUCTION

Great strides have been made in the past 35 years in diagnosing and treating women with breast cancer. Among the most important advances are the following:

- Mortality from breast cancer has declined almost 40% between 1989 and 2014, after having been unchanged for the 50 preceding years.

- In January 2018, there were more than 3.1 million women in the United States (U.S.) who had or have had breast cancer (Breastcancer.org).

- An estimated 40,610 women died from breast cancer in 2017, according to American Cancer Society (ACS) facts and figures.

- In 2018, an estimated 266,120 new invasive and 63,960 new noninvasive (in-situ) cancers were diagnosed (ACS estimates).

- At least 75% of women diagnosed with breast cancer are at average risk for breast cancer—that is, they have no other risk factors apart from increasing age and being female.

- For women at average risk, the lifetime risk for developing breast cancer is 1 in 8 (12%) (2006 to 2008 Surveillance, Epidemiology, and End Results [SEER] data); their mean age at diagnosis is 62 years.

- 5% to 10% of breast cancers are linked to genetic mutations.

- One out of every six breast cancers is diagnosed in women in their 40s.

- 40% of years of life lost are in women diagnosed with breast cancer in their 40s.

- 30% of breast cancers could be missed in women who skip just one annual mammogram during their 50s.

- At diagnosis, 62% of breast cancers are localized.

- At diagnosis, 31% of cancers have spread to regional (axillary) lymph nodes.

SURVIVAL FACTS (SEER, 2007 to 2013)

Stage of Cancer	Five-Year Relative Survival
Localized breast cancer (confined to breast)	99%
Regional metastases (spread to same side axillary lymph nodes)	85.2%
Distant metastases	26.9%

BREAST CANCER RISK FACTORS

The greatest risks for breast cancer are increasing age and being female. In the absence of other than these two factors, the risk for breast cancer increases from one in 229 women in their 30s, to 1 in 68 women in their 40s, to 1 in 37 women in their 50s, and to 1 in 26 women over 60 years of age (American Cancer Society). This corresponds to a 1-in-8 (12%) lifetime risk if a woman lives to be 70. Only 1% of breast cancer diagnoses occur in men.

A lifetime risk for breast cancer above 20% is considered to be high risk. Women with more than one first-degree relative diagnosed with breast cancer or ovarian cancer are at high risk. Women who have tested positive for the BRCA 1 or BRCA 2 genetic mutation or who have a first-degree relative who is a known BRCA carrier also are at high risk (up to an 85% lifetime risk). Survivors of Hodgkin's lymphoma who received high doses of radiation (more than 4 Gy) to the mediastinum are at high risk for radiation-induced breast cancer (35% by age 40, in one study) beginning eight years later (Bhatia, 1996). Some rare genetic syndromes—including Cowden's (PTEN gene), Li Fraumeni (the p53 gene), and Peutz-Jeghers syndrome (STK11 gene)—also are associated with an elevated risk for breast cancer.

In addition, several histopathologies discovered on breast needle core biopsy are benign but represent an increased risk for developing breast cancer: these are lobular neoplasia (atypical lobular hyperplasia [ALH] and lobular carcinoma *in situ* [LCIS]) and atypical ductal hyperplasia [ADH]).

Other factors that carry a mildly increased relative risk for developing breast cancer are nulliparity, first pregnancy at greater than age 30, early menarche (younger than age 12), late menopause (greater than age 55), and never having breastfed. None of these represents a significant risk alone, but each makes a small contribution to overall individual risk.

After age 35, Caucasian women have a higher risk for breast cancer than African-American women; in contrast, in the under-35 age group, African-American women have a slightly higher incidence. Mortality from breast cancer is higher among African-American women. Both incidence and mortality are lower for other racial and ethnic groups, including Hispanic and Asian women.

In addition to the major risk factors discussed above, some factors have been identified that confer so-called minor—and modifiable—risks for breast cancer. These include obesity, lack of exercise, excessive alcohol intake, and heavy smoking. Hormone replacement therapy (HRT) with combined estrogen and synthetic progestins also increases the risk for breast cancer (Campagnoli, 2005; Samson, 2016; and Morch, 2017), whereas estrogen-only HRT may not increase the risk. Additionally, HRT combining estrogen with natural progesterone does not appear to increase the risk of breast cancer (de Lignieres, 2002, and Fournier, 2005). As research continues regarding breast cancer risk, additional factors may be identified. For example, disruption of normal sleep patterns—such as working the night shift—has been discussed as a possible breast cancer risk factor (Xuelei, 2018).

EARLY DETECTION AT THE EARLIEST STAGE

The earliest stage (stage 0) of breast cancer is ductal carcinoma *in situ* (DCIS)—that is, abnormal cells confined by the basement membrane of the terminal duct lobule, which is the basic anatomic unit of the breast. The standard of care for the treatment of DCIS is surgical excision with clear margins, followed by whole or partial breast irradiation. If the tumor is estrogen-receptor (ER) –positive and the patient is premenopausal, an estrogen receptor antagonist, such as tamoxifen, is given for five to ten years. For postmenopausal women with ER-positive tumors, the recommendation is for postsurgical treatment with an aromatase inhibitor for five years. When these protocols are followed, survival after DCIS is almost 100%.

Between 1973 and 1990, the incidence of DCIS increased by a factor of seven; before 1985, DCIS accounted for fewer than 5% of breast cancer diagnoses. The incidence increased after the introduction and widespread acceptance of mammography screening and, since 1998, 20% to 30% of cancers diagnosed are DCIS. For every four invasive breast cancer diagnoses, there is one DCIS, especially over the age of 50. By the year 2020, more than one million women in the U.S. will be living with a past diagnosis of DCIS.

SCREENING GUIDELINES AND CONTROVERSIES

Since the advent of regular breast cancer screening in the mid-1980s, mortality from breast cancer—which had remained constant for the prior 50 years—has decreased by almost 40%. Thus, the life-saving benefits of screening are clear; less clear are issues regarding timing: when should screening begin and how often should it be done?

Screening Mammography: Average-Risk Women

For screening average-risk women, the most common recommendation is annual mammography starting at 40 years of age. This guideline is endorsed by the American College of Obstetricians and Gynecologists (ACOG) and the American College of Radiology (ACR). The American Cancer Society recommends annual screening beginning at age 45. The American College of Physicians (ACP) recommends annual mammography at 50 years of age and older, with clinicians performing individualized assessments for breast cancer risk to help guide decisions about screening mammography for women between 40 and 49 years of age; the ACP recognizes that this approach remains "a challenge" (Qaseem, 2007).

The U.S. Preventive Services Task Force (USPSTF) recommendations are controversial. As of January 2016, the USPSTF recommends biennial screening mammography for women from 50 to 74 years of age. Before age 50, the USPSTF recommends individualized decision-making. "The decision to start screening mammography in women prior to age 50 should be an individual one. Women who place a higher value on the potential benefit than the potential harms may choose to begin biennial screening between the ages of 40 and 49 years."

Screening mammography is covered without co-pay or deductible under the

Affordable Care Act of 2010. Currently, it is covered annually after the age of 40. There is no upper age limit. The USPSTF has drafted a recommendation which may change ages and frequency. However, the Protecting Access to Lifesaving Screenings (PALS) Act has passed a moratorium on any changes until January of 2019.

Screening Mammography:
Intermediate- and High-Risk Patients

Intermediate risk, defined as lifetime risk between 15% and 20%, includes a personal history of breast or ovarian cancer, a prior breast biopsy showing atypical ductal hyperplasia or atypical lobular hyperplasia, or multiple relatives with breast cancer who were not premenopausal at the time of diagnosis (premenopausal cancer in a first-degree relative is a significant risk).

There are no guidelines for screening intermediate-risk women, although there is an awareness by breast imagers of the need for greater scrutiny. Many will add whole breast ultrasound for intermediate-risk women who have increased breast density (Berg, 2012, and ACR, 2017). (For additional information on the Appropriateness Criteria methodology and other supporting documents go to www.acr.org/ac).

Women considered at high risk should have annual screening mammograms and contrast-enhanced breast magnetic resonance imaging (MRI) beginning ten years earlier than the youngest age at which cancer was diagnosed in their relative(s). Young women who had radiation therapy to the chest or mediastinum for lymphoma should start receiving mammograms eight years after the radiation. Intermediate-risk patients do not qualify for MRI screening because insurance companies usually only cover this test for high-risk patients (Lee, 2010, and ACR, 2017).

BREAST IMAGING BEYOND MAMMOGRAPHY

Mammography represents an important advance in early breast cancer detection. Mammographic sensitivity—that is, the proportion of cancers visualized—ranges from less than 50 in 85% depending on degree of breast density. In some cases, the results of initial studies may be equivocal—for example, higher breast density in younger women, normal asymmetries in breasts, and common benign findings— repeat examinations (recalls) may be requested.

Additional imaging may resolve the question of a possible malignancy. A biopsy is performed if malignancy cannot be ruled out for an apparent abnormality seen on a mammogram. A false-positive mammogram is one where a possible abnormality proved normal or benign on additional imaging. The term false positive is also used when a biopsy performed for a suspicious finding results in benign pathology, i.e., no malignancy is present. The majority of biopsies done following mammography (70% to-80%) are benign and therefore are considered false positive. But this is good news for the patient.

- The chance of a recall examination after routine screening is one in ten (although it may be higher after the first mammogram, because there is no previous examination to which it can be compared).

- The chance of a needle biopsy (performed by the radiologist specializing in breast imaging) after a recall examination, is one in five of those recalled.

- The chance of the biopsy being benign is four out of five; only one in five biopsies will demonstrate a malignancy.

- To summarize, if 1,000 women are screened, 100 may be recalled, and 20 out of 1,000 may be biopsied, but only five will have cancer.

After the recall, sometimes mammographers suggest a "short-interval follow-up," usually in six months; this would be the recommendation for these patients if the expected chance of malignancy is calculated to be less than 2%. This sometimes happens when the findings are calcifications, asymmetries, or probable fibroadenomas in young women. However, the short-interval follow-up is suggested only after a full evaluation, including extra views and, occasionally, the addition of ultrasound. It is only by carefully pursuing potential abnormalities that mammographers can pick up the earliest cancers.

About 40% of women in the U.S. have dense breast tissue on their mammogram, making mammography less sensitive and possibly obscuring small masses. Dense breast tissue also represents an independent risk factor for breast cancer. Multiple states have mandated patient notification in a "Lay letter" if the mammogram shows dense breast tissue. This is to increase a woman's awareness that breast density is an issue for her and also to inform her that supplemental imaging is available.

Tomosynthesis (3D Mammography)

Tomosynthesis, also referred to as 3D mammography, was developed to overcome some of the disadvantages of dense breasts causing false-positive results and mammography recalls. The first manufacturer (Hologic) received approval for this device from the U.S. Food and Drug Administration in 2011; other devices were approved subsequently.

The tomosynthesis examination, consisting of two views with compression, is performed at the same time as the conventional mammogram. The images are then reconstructed for "3D" viewing at the work station. The tomosynthesis examination—essentially, two mammograms—requires more time than the conventional mammogram and increases radiation exposure. Gradually, mammography practices are performing the tomosynthesis portion of the examination without the conventional mammogram, reducing the radiation dose to that equivalent to a 2D mammogram.

Tomosynthesis use has resulted in a reduction in callbacks due to overlapping tissue. At the same time, the literature shows that this technique has resulted in the detection of smaller cancers, making tomosynthesis a better mammogram for dense breasts (Destounis, 2015, and Sharpe, 2016).

Screening with Breast Ultrasound

Because dense breasts are associated with a four- to six-fold increased risk for breast cancer (Harvey, 2004), whole breast ultrasound is recommended as additional screening for mammographically dense breasts in three states (Connecticut, Texas, and Virginia). In women with dense breasts, a negative mammogram, and a normal clinical examination, the addition of breast ultrasound detects an additional 2.8 to 4.6 breast cancers per 1,000 women (Berg, 2008). However, the ultrasound examination is time-consuming, operator-dependent, and results in more false-positive findings (that is, biopsies with a benign final result) than mammography alone.

Other Screening Technologies

Several other screening techniques have been developed but currently are not in general use.

- Thermography: <u>Not</u> recommended (sensitivity only 43%) (Beahrs, 1979).

- Molecular imaging: Associated with a high radiation dose (Hendrick, 2010). Not appropriate for annual screening. This also is known as breast-specific gamma imaging and uses the isotope Tc 99m sestimibi.

- Positron-emission tomography (PET) and positron-emission mammography (PEM) using fluoro-deoxyglucose (FDG).

Breast specific gamma imaging and PET provide very high radiation exposure and are not sensitive for DCIS. Breast-specific gamma imaging has been proposed as a technique for screening. Positron-emission tomography usually is reserved for staging after a diagnosis of invasive cancer with possible metastatic spread.

CONCLUSION

Obstetrics and Gynecology providers often serve as the only primary care provider for women between the ages of 18 and 80. Because breast cancer will affect one in eight women, annual breast screening should begin after age 40, with special consideration for those at high risk based on personal or family history. Supplemental imaging with ultrasound should be offered to women with dense breasts. Patients have many questions and concerns regarding breast cancer and the role of breast screening. The OB/GYN care provider must be knowledgeable about this area of health and also be sensitive to the emotional impact presented by this disease.

For additional information, refer to the following websites:
www.mammographysaveslives.org/
http://areyoudenseadvocacy.org/dense/
www.breastcancer.org

REFERENCES

1. American College of Radiology ACR Appropriateness Criteria® Breast Cancer Screening (revised 2017). https://acsearch.acr.org/docs/70910/Narrative/

2. American Cancer Society. <u>Breast Cancer Facts and Figures</u>, 2017. Atlanta: American Cancer Society.

3. Beahrs OH, Shapiror S, and Smart CR (1979). Summary report of the working group to review the National Cancer Institute-American Cancer Society Breast Cancer Detection Demonstration Projects. Journal of the National Cancer Institute, 62(3):641-650.

4. Berg WA, Blume JD, Cormack JB, Mendelson EB, Lehrer D, Böhm-Vélez M, Pisano ED, Jong RA, Evans WP, Morton MJ, Mahoney MC, Larsen LH, Barr RG, Farria DM, Marques HS, and Boparai; ACRIN 6666 Investigators (2008). Combined screening with ultrasound and mammography vs. mammography alone in women at elevated risk of breast cancer. Journal of the American Medical Association, 299(18):2151-2163.

5. Berg WA, Zhang Z, Lehrer D, Jong RA, Pisano ED, Barr RG, Böhm-Vélez M, Mahoney MC, Evans WP 3rd, Larsen LH, Morton MJ, Mendelson EB, Farria DM, Cormack JB, Marques HS, Adams A, Yeh NM, and Gabrielli G (2012). Detection of breast cancer with addition of annual screening ultrasound or a single screening MRI to mammography in women with elevated breast cancer risk. JAMA, 307(13):1394-1404.

6. Bhatia S, Robison LL, Oberlin O, Greenberg M, Bunin G, Fossati-Bellani F, and Meadow A (1996). Breast Cancer and other second neoplasm after childhood Hodgkin's disease. The New England Journal of Medicine, 334:745-752.

7. Boyd NF, Guo H, Martin LJ, Sun L, Stones J, Fishell E, Jong R, Hislop G, Chiarelli A, Minkin S, and Yaffe M (2007). Mammographic density and the risk and detection of breast cancer. The New England Journal of Medicine, 356:227–236. http://www.breastcancer.org/symptoms/understand_bc/statistics

8. Campagnoli C, Clavel-Chapelon F, Kaake R, Peris C, and Berrino F (2005). Progestins and progesterone in hormone replacement therapy and the risk of breast cancer. Journal of Steroid Biochemistry and Molecular Biology, 96(2):95-108.

9. Crystal P, Strano SD, Shcharynski S, and Koretz MJ (2003). Using sonography to screen women with mammographically dense breasts. AJR. American Journal of Roentgenology, 181:177–182.

10. de Lignieres B (2002). Effects of progestogens on the postmenopausal breast. Climacteric, 5(3):229-235.

11. Destounis SV, Morgan R, and Arieno A (2015). Screening for dense breasts: Digital breast tomosynthesis. American Journal of Roentgenology, 204(2):261-264.

12. Fournier A, Berrino F, Riboli E, Avenel V, and Clavel-Chapelon F (2005). Breast cancer risk in relation to different types of hormone replacement therapy in the E3N-EPIC cohort. International Journal of Cancer, 114(3):448-454.

13. Harvey JA and Bovbjerg VE (2004). Quantitative assessment of mammographic breast density relationship with breast cancer risk: Relationship with breast cancer risk. Radiology, 230:29-41.

14. Hendrick RE (2010). Radiation doses and cancer risks from breast imaging studies. Radiology, 257(1):246-53.

15. Howlader N, Noone AM, Krapcho M, Miller D, Bishop K, Kosary CL, Yu M, Ruhl J, Tatalovich Z, Mariotto A, Lewis DR, Chen HS, Feuer EJ, Cronin KA (eds). SEER Cancer Statistics Review, 1975-2014, National Cancer Institute. Bethesda, MD, https://seer.cancer.gov/csr/1975_2014, based on November 2016 SEER data submission, posted

to the SEER web site, April 2017.

16. Kaplan SS (2001). Clinical utility of bilateral whole-breast US in the evaluation of women with dense breast tissue. Radiology, 221:641–664.

17. Kolb TM, Lichy J, and Newhouse JH (2002). Comparison of the performance of screening mammography, physical examination, and breast US and evaluation of factors that influence them: An analysis of 27,825 patient evaluations. Radiology, 225:165–175.

18. Lee CH, Dershaw DD, Kopans D, Evans P, Monsees B, Monticciolo D, Brenner RJ, Bassett L, Berg W, Feig S, Hendrick E, Mendelson E, D'Orsi C, Sickles E, and Burhenne LW (2010). Breast cancer screening with imaging: Recommendations from the Society of Breast Imaging and the ACR on the use of mammography, breast MRI, breast ultrasound, and other technologies for the detection of clinically occult breast cancer. Journal of the American College of Radiology, 7(1):18-27.

19. Morch LS, Skovlund CW, Hannaford PC, Iversen L, Fielding S, and Lidegaard O (2017). Contemporary hormone contraception and the risk of breast cancer. New England Journal of Medicine, 37:2228-2239.

20. Qaseem A, Snow V, Sherif K, Aronson M, Weiss K, and Owens D (2007). Screening mammography for women 40 to 49 years of age: A clinical practice guideline from the american college of physicians. Annals of Internal Medicine, 147:511-515.

21. Samson M, Porter N, Orekoya O, Hebert JR, Adams SA, Bennet CL, and Steck SE (2016). Progestin and breast cancer risk: A systematic review. Breast Cancer Res and Treatment, 155(1):3-12.

22. Screening for Breast Cancer: U.S preventive Services Task Force Recommendation Statement (2009). Annals of Internal Medicine, 151:716-726.

23. Sharpe RE Jr, Venkataraman S, Phillips J, Dialani V, Fein-Zachary VJ, Prakash S, Slanetz PJ, and Mehta TS (2016). Increased cancer detection rate and variations in the recall rate resulting from implementation of 3D digital breast tomosynthesis into a population-based screening program. Radiology, 278(3):698-706.

24. Surveillance, Epidemiology and End Results (SEER) 2001-2007. National Cancer Institute.

25. Trivedi AN, Leyva B, Lee Y, Panagiotou OA, and Dahabreh IJ (2018). Elimination of cost sharing for screening mammography in Medicare Advantage Plans. New England Journal of Medicine, 378:262-269.

26. U.S. Preventive services task force (USPSTF).

27. Xuelei (2018). Night shift work increases the risks of multiple primary cancers in women: A systematic review and meta-analysis of 61 articles. Cancer Epidemiology, Biomarkers, and Prevention, 27(1):25-40.

BREAST CANCER GENETICS

Audrey L. Schroeder, M.S. and Kelly Q. Minks, M.S.

INTRODUCTION

Nearly all women have thought about breast cancer and whether they could be at risk. Many have wondered, "What is my specific risk to develop breast cancer?", "When do I need to start screening for breast cancer?", and "What is the best way to screen for breast cancer?" For some women, often due to a personal experience with breast cancer themselves or with a close family member or friend who has been affected, there may be additional questions like, "What caused the development of this breast cancer?", "What is the chance of developing another breast cancer or some other type of cancer in the future?", and "Could this be genetic?" In this chapter, we will explore the area of breast cancer genetics and some situations in which an individual's breast cancer may be "genetic."

To start, there is a distinction between using the terms "genetic" and "hereditary" when discussing the cause of breast cancer. All types of cancers, including breast cancer, are technically "genetic," as they are caused by genetic changes, also known as mutations (or pathogenic variants), within the genes of a cell. If mutations develop and accumulate within critical regions of the genes, this can cause that cell to begin dividing at a rapid and uncontrollable rate. That cell can then become a cancer. Typically, these mutations are acquired over an individual's lifetime (and are not present at birth), occurring as sporadic (random) events and/or as the result of environmental exposures. When cancers are examined at a molecular level, the specific genetic mutations within that cancer can be identified. Sometimes an individual's physician may order specialized testing to identify which specific mutations exist in the cancer or tumor, as this can give information about prognosis and the most effective treatment, particularly in decisions about chemotherapy.

When a cancer is "hereditary," it means that an individual was born with a gene mutation that increases his or her lifetime risk of developing one or more types of cancer. Approximately 5% to 10% of all breast cancers are "hereditary." Typically, in individuals who have "hereditary" forms of breast cancer, an inherited mutation can be identified in a blood sample. In these same individuals, we would expect their breast tumor to have the same mutation as well as additional gene mutations that have been acquired during the development of the tumor.

A hereditary form of breast cancer may be suspected in a family if there are multiple generations in the family who are affected with breast cancer, suggesting that an inherited mutation is being passed down from parent to offspring. Other "red flags" also may be present, prompting genetic evaluation. These will be explored later in the chapter.

The most well-known and common breast cancer genes (BRCA) are the BRCA1 and BRCA2 genes. Many people have become familiar with these genes over the past several years, as awareness about genetic testing has increased and as testing becomes more available. In 1990, Dr. Mary-Claire King demonstrated that a hypothetical gene (later to be named BRCA1) on chromosome 17 was linked to early-onset familial breast cancers. In the years that followed, the BRCA2 gene also was discovered, and more information about the location and makeup of these genes was characterized. Commercial clinical DNA testing of the BRCA1 and BRCA2 genes was first offered in 1996 by Myriad Genetic Laboratories. Myriad Genetic Laboratories performed all clinical testing of the BRCA1 and BRCA2 genes in the United States (U.S.) until the 2013 Supreme Court ruled that naturally occurring genes may not be patented (Hurst, 2014). Currently, several clinical laboratories in the U.S. offer BRCA1 and BRCA2 genetic testing.

The number of women (and men) who undergo BRCA1 and BRCA2 genetic testing continues to increase. Our knowledge of hereditary breast cancer genes and genetic testing technology also has continued to evolve and advance over the years. One major advancement is that researchers now have identified several other genes that can cause hereditary forms of breast cancer. Another major advancement is that newer DNA testing technology, called next generation sequencing or massively parallel sequencing, has become available, which allows laboratories to analyze multiple genes at once within a short timeframe and at a relatively low cost. These factors have contributed to the growing use of multi-gene hereditary cancer panels in which a laboratory can perform DNA testing of multiple cancer genes at once. When these multi-gene panels are ordered for the purpose of evaluating hereditary breast cancer risk, they typically include the BRCA1 and BRCA2 genes as well as additional cancer susceptibility genes such as the ATM, CHEK2, and PALB2 genes, to name a few.

All individuals have the BRCA1 and BRCA2 genes, as well as other genes associated with hereditary breast cancer, in their cells. Each individual typically has two copies of the BRCA1 gene (one inherited from each parent) and two copies of the BRCA2 gene (also with one inherited from each parent). The BRCA1 and BRCA2 genes have significant roles in the cells, making proteins that help to maintain normal DNA repair and cell growth and division (NCCN, 2017, and GeneReviews, 2017). Thus, when working normally, they provide a level of protection against certain types of cancer such as breast cancer and ovarian cancer. When an individual has an inherited mutation in the BRCA1 or BRCA2 gene, the protein that the gene typically forms is not working properly or at all. This causes that individual to be more susceptible to certain types of cancers, and he or she is considered to have a significantly increased risk for developing cancer.

For a woman who has an inherited BRCA1 or BRCA2 gene mutation, her highest risks are for the development of breast and ovarian cancer, including ovarian-related cancers such as primary peritoneal cancer and fallopian tube cancer. This is why individuals with a BRCA1 or BRCA2 mutation are sometimes described as having "Hereditary Breast and Ovarian Cancer Syndrome," or "HBOC." BRCA1 and BRCA2 gene mutations also are associated with increased risks for other cancer types, although to a lesser extent in terms of lifetime risk. Men with BRCA1 and BRCA2 mutations are at increased risk for prostate cancer and male breast cancer, particularly if they have a BRCA2 mutation. Men and women also are suspected to have increased risk for other cancers such as pancreatic cancer and melanoma, particularly with BRCA2 mutations. There still is more information that we expect to learn over time about BRCA1- and BRCA2-associated cancer risks, including clarification on whether there also may be increased risk for endometrial cancer, leukemia, colorectal cancer, or others.

For women who have inherited BRCA1 or BRCA2 mutations but who have never had cancer, their estimated lifetime breast cancer risk falls within the range of approximately 46% to 87% (Petrucelli, 2016). This is a dramatically increased risk when compared to the general population lifetime risk for breast cancer of approximately 12.4% (NIH SEERa). For women with a BRCA1 or BRCA2 mutation who have already had a breast cancer, they also are considered at increased risk for a second new breast cancer referred to as a new "primary" cancer compared to women without a BRCA1 or BRCA2 gene mutation.

Due to these significantly increased risks for breast cancer, there are several medical management and screening considerations that are discussed when a woman tests positive for a mutation. For women with a mutation who are newly diagnosed with breast cancer, bilateral mastectomy may be considered as a primary surgical treatment because of their increased risk for a second primary breast cancer. However, a genetic test result is not the only factor that influences surgical and treatment recommendations. Unaffected women with a mutation also may consider prophylactic mastectomy to reduce their risk for breast cancer. Another option is taking an oral medication, such as tamoxifen, to reduce breast cancer risk. For unaffected women who have not elected to proceed with risk-reducing mastectomy and for women with breast cancer who have proceeded with conservative management (i.e., lumpectomy), enhanced breast cancer screening is critical. Per the 2017 National Comprehensive Cancer Network (NCCN) guidelines, it usually is recommended that a BRCA-positive woman begin breast cancer screening starting at approximately age 25. Occasionally, it is recommended that a woman begin even earlier if there is a family member who was diagnosed at a very young age. Breast cancer screening typically involves clinical breast examinations every six to 12 months starting at age 25, annual breast magnetic resonance imaging (MRI) starting at age 25, and annual breast MRI combined with annual mammogram starting at age 30. When mammogram is implemented at age 30, most medical centers alternate between mammogram and breast MRI so that women have one of these breast imaging studies every six months. Breast awareness is important for all women, and women should report any changes in their breasts promptly to their healthcare providers.

For women who have inherited BRCA1 or BRCA2 mutations but who have never had cancer, their estimated lifetime ovarian cancer risk falls within the range of approximately 16.5% to 63% (Petrucelli, 2016). This is a significantly increased risk when compared to the general population lifetime risk for ovarian cancer of approximately 1.3% (NIH SEERb). Due to the significantly higher risk of ovarian cancer for women with mutations, and because there is not an effective screening method for detection of ovarian cancer, risk-reducing surgery is recommended in these cases. (This is in contrast to breast cancer surgical options in which risk-reducing mastectomy is a "consideration" rather than a "recommendation"). The

2017 NCCN guidelines recommend that risk-reducing salpingo-oophorectomy (removal of fallopian tubes and ovaries) typically be performed between 35 and 40 years of age and upon completion of childbearing. Not only does this surgery significantly reduce risk for ovarian cancer, it also provides some risk reduction for the development of breast cancer (NCCN, 2017). As BRCA2-associated ovarian cancers may occur at older ages than BRCA1-associated ovarian cancers, it is reasonable to delay risk-reducing salpingo-oophorectomy until 45 to 50 years of age in patients with BRCA2 mutations who have already maximized their breast cancer prevention (i.e., undergone bilateral mastectomy). Women who have not undergone risk-reducing salpingo-oophorectomy can consider ovarian cancer "screening," with an understanding that these methods have not been proven to be effective in detecting early-stage ovarian cancer. This may include having annual transvaginal ultrasounds (sonograms) and a CA-125 tumor marker blood test starting at 30 to 35 years of age. Separately, studies have shown that oral contraceptive use can reduce risk for ovarian cancer in women who have BRCA1 and BRCA2 gene mutations (Rebbeck, 2002, and NCCN, 2017). There has been conflicting data as to whether oral contraceptive use increases risk for breast cancer in women who have mutations (NCCN, 2017).

In addition to understanding their own cancer risks, the majority of individuals who undergo genetic testing also are interested in learning about whether their family members could be at risk for the mutation. For the majority of known hereditary breast cancer genes, including BRCA1 and BRCA2, if a mutation is identified, other family members are at risk. To better understand these risks, it is important to know that most individuals who test positive for a BRCA1 or BRCA2 mutation are found to have a mutation in just one of these genes. Very rarely is an individual identified with a mutation in both the BRCA1 and BRCA2 gene. Further, individuals with a BRCA1 or BRCA2 mutation are born with just one mutation on one copy of the gene, while the other copy of the gene is normal. This is known as being heterozygous for a gene mutation. (Note that there are other genetic syndromes and conditions that result from having two mutations, with one mutation on each copy of a gene. This is known as being homozygous.) Usually, the mutation has been inherited from one of that individual's parents; however, the most common testing techniques cannot tell us from which parent it came. If an individual with a BRCA1 mutation has children, he or she will pass one of those BRCA1 genes down to each child: either the gene with the mutation or the gene without the mutation. Therefore, each child has a one in two chance, or an approximate 50% likelihood, of having the BRCA1 mutation. The same inheritance pattern, which is described as an autosomal dominant inheritance pattern, also is observed with BRCA2 gene mutations. In evaluating risks for other family members, we know that since these mutations almost always are inherited from a parent, each parent has up to a 50% chance of having the mutation. In addition, an individual's siblings will have up to a 50% chance of having the mutation. Other family members such as aunts, uncles, nieces, nephews, and cousins also may be at risk of having the mutation. If a mutation is identified in an individual, it is very common that other

> **As of 2017, breast density notification laws were in place in 30 states.**
>
> **The Affordable Care Act (ACA) eliminated co-pays and deductibles for screening mammography, resulting in increased rate of screening (Trivedi, 2018).**

family members will be interested in genetic testing to determine if they also have the mutation. Testing for them can determine whether they have or have not inherited that mutation. This allows them and their physicians to understand whether they also are at significantly increased risk for cancer.

WHO SHOULD BE TESTED?

So who should be thinking about BRCA1 and BRCA2 genetic testing to determine if they have, or are at risk for, a hereditary form of cancer? As it currently stands in the U.S., not all women are considered candidates for genetic testing. Although some experts in the medical genetics community have proposed general population testing of the BRCA1 and BRCA2 genes, this currently is not the standard approach. Current testing guidelines such as those developed by the NCCN, The American Society of Breast Surgeons, The American College of Obstetricians and Gynecologists, The Society of Gynecologic Oncologists, and others, provide genetic testing criteria that can be used by healthcare providers to determine which patients have a significantly increased risk for a mutation and should be offered testing. Although there can be several nuances in evaluating an individual's risk for a mutation (such as size of the family and whether there is a preponderance of males), some of the most common criteria include the following.

- The individual is from a family with a known gene mutation.

- An individual is diagnosed with "early-onset" breast cancer (typically defined as being diagnosed at age 45 years or under, or age 50 years or under, depending upon the guideline), regardless of family history.

- An individual diagnosed with breast cancer at age 60 or under if the breast cancer is "triple negative." This is due to our understanding that patients with "triple-negative" breast cancers (tumors characterized as estrogen-receptor [ER]-/progesterone-receptor [PR]-negative and human epidermal growth factor receptor 2 [HER2]-negative) are more likely to have a mutation, particularly a BRCA1 mutation (NCCN, 2017)

- An individual with breast cancer at any age and with additional family history of cancer such as a close relative with ovarian cancer, a close male relative with breast cancer, or two or more close blood relatives with breast cancer, pancreatic cancer, or prostate cancer (specifically more aggressive prostate cancer, with a Gleason score of 7 or higher) at any age.

- An individual with breast cancer at any age who is of Ashkenazi Jewish ancestry. This is a criterion due to the higher prevalence of BRCA1 and BRCA2 gene mutations in individuals of Ashkenazi Jewish ancestry compared to the prevalence of mutations observed in individuals who are not Ashkenazi Jewish.

- An individual with ovarian cancer diagnosed at any age.

- A male with breast cancer at any age.

- An unaffected individual (who has never had cancer) who has a significant family history of breast cancer, ovarian cancer, male breast cancer, pancreatic cancer, or prostate cancer such as that noted above.

Note that this is not an exhaustive list of all possible testing criteria.

PERFORMING A CANCER RISK ASSESSMENT

The process of undergoing a cancer risk assessment and genetic testing should involve a few key components, including both pre-test counseling and post-test counseling. During pre-test counseling, the healthcare provider should collect a comprehensive medical and family history, establish and communicate with the patient the differential diagnosis (i.e., which hereditary cancer syndromes, if any, are most likely), and facilitate the informed consent process for genetic testing. This includes review of the benefits, risks, limitations, and alternatives to genetic testing. Individuals should be prepared for possible outcomes of genetic testing including the possibilities of a positive result (mutation identified which confirms hereditary cancer risk), negative result (no mutation identified), or uncertain result (a variant or change in the gene is identified, but it is unknown if this causes an increased risk for cancer) and how these results might be interpreted in terms of level of cancer risk and screening and medical management recommendations. The opportunity for an individual to have his or her specific questions addressed, such as those relating to topics such as genetic discrimination or potential genetic risks to family members, also should be provided. Post-test counseling typically incudes discussion of genetic test results interpreted in the context of that patient's individual and family medical history. That individual's level of cancer risk is discussed, along with recommended cancer screening and medical management. Post-test counseling also usually involves discussions about genetic testing for at-risk relatives and, particularly if positive for a mutation, provision of resources including information about the specific cancer syndrome, support group resources, and potential research studies. Some individuals also require psychologic support (NCCN, 2017). The following vignettes illustrate some common scenarios that occur during the process of a cancer risk assessment.

Vignette #1: Woman Diagnosed with Breast Cancer who Tests Positive for BRCA Gene Mutation

Ana is a 40-year-old female who recently was found to have an infiltrating ductal carcinoma, ER+/PR+/HER2-, of her left breast after feeling a lump while doing a self-breast examination. At her first appointment with the breast surgeon, genetic testing was recommended for Ana based on her young age of diagnosis.

Ana's surgeon let Ana know that sometimes genetic testing can help with surgical decision-making and placed a referral for her to see a genetic counselor. Within the same week, Ana and her husband met with a genetic counselor for pre-test counseling.

Ana started off the counseling session by saying that she had heard about genetic testing through a friend whose mother had ovarian cancer. Her friend's mother tested positive for a mutation in the BRCA1 gene, but her friend had tested negative. A detailed, three-generation family history is taken from Ana and, while her family was very small, there are no other family members with a history of breast or other cancers. Ana tells the genetic counselor that she previously had been healthy; she had no major medical problems and no history of other cancers. The genetic counselor also asks Ana if she has ever had a surgery to remove either of her ovaries or her uterus, which she has not. Ana and her husband have one ten-year-old daughter who is in good health, and they are not planning to have more children.

The genetic counselor then reviews the current guidelines for genetic testing for hereditary breast cancer with Ana. The counselor reviews some of the characteristics seen more commonly in individuals and families with inherited breast cancer such as young age of onset and multiple generations with cancer. She explains that genetic testing guidelines are in place to help determine which individuals or families have an increased chance of having a hereditary breast cancer and, therefore, who would benefit from testing. Ana met the genetic testing criteria, because she had a young onset of breast cancer, but the counselor explains that it does not mean her breast cancer is definitely hereditary.

The counselor provides Ana with information about the percentage of breast cancers that are hereditary and the most common genes associated with hereditary breast cancer, BRCA1 and BRCA2. Ana has an upcoming appointment with a plastic surgeon, and her breast surgery had been scheduled in three weeks. The counselor reviews with Ana that if she tests positive for a BRCA1 or BRCA2 gene mutation, not only would it confirm this as the hereditary cause for her breast cancer, but it would also indicate significantly increased risk for a second primary breast cancer. For this reason, one benefit of genetic testing for mutations in the BRCA1 and BRCA2 genes is to assist with surgical decision-making. Women

53

who have a BRCA1 or a BRCA2 gene mutation are found to be at an increased risk for a second primary breast cancer in the opposite breast (contralateral breast cancer) and some studies also find an increased risk for a second primary breast cancer in the same breast (ipsilateral breast cancer). The risk for women with BRCA1 gene mutations for contralateral breast cancer is estimated to be as high as 83% and the risk for women with BRCA2 mutations for contralateral breast cancer is estimated to be as high as 62% (Mavaddat, 2013). Therefore, many women who are found to have a BRCA1 or a BRCA2 gene mutation may choose to have a bilateral mastectomy versus having a breast-conserving surgery (i.e., lumpectomy) in order to reduce their risk of developing a second primary breast cancer. Ana states that she already is nervous about getting breast cancer again and would consider having a bilateral mastectomy instead of a lumpectomy if she is found to have a BRCA1 or BRCA2 gene mutation.

The genetic counselor also discusses that, in addition to a higher risk for a second primary breast cancer, women who have a BRCA1 or a BRCA2 gene mutation also are at increased risk for ovarian cancer. The genetic counselor reviews the recommendation that women who have a BRCA1 or BRCA2 gene mutation consider a risk-reducing salpingo-oophorectomy between the ages of 35 and 40 and after childbearing. In addition to reducing risk for ovarian cancer, a risk-reducing salpingo-oophorectomy is thought to reduce the risk for developing breast cancer (Rebbeck, 2002). Ana states that she is done having children and, if necessary, would consider this surgery to reduce her chance of developing ovarian cancer.

Ana expresses concern for her daughter's risk of having a BRCA1 or BRCA2 gene mutation if she tests positive. The genetic counselor talks with Ana about the inheritance of mutations in the BRCA1 and BRCA2 genes. Because mutations in the BRCA1 and BRCA2 genes are inherited in an autosomal dominant pattern, Ana's daughter would have a 50% chance of inheriting the same mutation. If Ana tests negative for BRCA1 and BRCA2 mutations, Ana's daughter would not need to have genetic testing; however, she would still be at an increased risk for breast cancer based on the family history. If Ana tests negative for mutations in BRCA1 and BRCA2, Ana's daughter would be encouraged to pursue breast screening starting at age 30 to 35 (five to ten years younger than the earliest diagnosis in the family). The genetic counselor reassures Ana that her daughter still is very young, and that if Ana's genetic test result is positive for a mutation in the BRCA1 or BRCA2 genes, testing for her daughter would not be necessary until she is at least 18 years old when she can make an autonomous and informed decision. With that information, Ana feels better knowing that her daughter will receive earlier breast screening, even if Ana is not found to have a mutation in the BRCA1 or BRCA2 genes.

Due to the improvement in turnaround times for genetic testing, Ana returns for an in-person results disclosure appointment with the genetic counselor the week of her surgery. The genetic counselor now tells Ana that she was found to have a mutation in the BRCA1 gene. Ana's initial reaction is shock—she knew that it was a possibility for her to have positive genetic testing, but she still was hoping it would come back negative. Despite this, Ana states she feels she made the right choice to pursue testing, because she now will choose to have a bilateral mastectomy versus a lumpectomy given the increased risk for another breast cancer. She also expresses interest, following her breast cancer treatment, to discuss a risk-reducing salpingo-oophorectomy. Ana is encouraged to discuss this with her OB/GYN and is given a referral to a gynecologic oncologist in the area.

Vignette #2: Unaffected Young Woman who Tests Positive for a Familial BRCA Gene Mutation

Elizabeth is a healthy, 30-year-old female with a family history of breast cancer due to a BRCA2 gene mutation. She presents to a new gynecology office for a new patient visit and reviews the history with her doctor. Her gynecologist recommends that she see a genetic counselor to discuss and consider genetic testing. Elizabeth comes to the genetic counseling appointment alone.

The genetic counselor reviews Elizabeth's medical history and family history. Elizabeth has never had a mammogram and both her uterus and ovaries are intact. She has no children but is getting married in a year and is interested in having children in the future. Elizabeth's mother had a history of breast cancer diagnosed at age 41, her maternal grandmother was diagnosed with ovarian cancer at age 53, and her maternal uncle was diagnosed with pancreatic cancer at age 55. Elizabeth's mother recently had genetic testing, which indicated a mutation in the BRCA2 gene. Elizabeth says her mother has her genetic test report at home, but Elizabeth did not bring it with her to the appointment.

The counselor explains to Elizabeth that it is important to see the genetic test report before pursuing the genetic testing. This is to ensure that a mutation was identified in the BRCA2 gene, rather than a variant of uncertain significance or a benign variant. Additionally, it is important to confirm the specific mutation within the BRCA2 gene and to identify the laboratory where the original family member had testing. The counselor explains to Elizabeth that this allows the laboratory to test Elizabeth for only the mutation identified in her mother, rather than looking at the entire BRCA2 gene, which is not necessary in most cases. As there are slight differences in testing technology among laboratories, it also is preferable to send the sample to the same laboratory where the original family member had testing. Elizabeth calls her mother who faxes over a copy of the genetic test, which in fact shows a mutation in the BRCA2 gene.

After reviewing information about the BRCA2 gene and the associated risks for cancer, the counselor reviews Elizabeth's risk for inheriting the BRCA2 gene mutation, which is 50%. The genetic counselor reviews some of the screening and preventative options for women who are at an increased risk for breast cancer due to a BRCA2 gene mutation. Screening options include increased breast cancer screenings with clinical breast examinations, annual mammograms, and annual breast MRIs. Preventative options include risk-reducing mastectomy, with or without reconstruction, and chemoprevention using tamoxifen, an oral medication that has been shown to reduce risk for breast cancer in women who carry mutations. It is estimated that tamoxifen reduces the risk for breast cancer by 62% in unaffected women who have a BRCA2 gene mutation (King, 2001). The genetic counselor also discusses screening and preventative options for ovarian cancer. Elizabeth mentions that she is interested in having children after she gets married in a year. The counselor discusses with Elizabeth that because of the lack of effective screening options for ovarian cancer, the recommendation in women with BRCA1 and BRCA2 gene mutations is to pursue risk-reducing salpingo-oophorectomy between the ages of 35 and 40 and after childbearing. Lastly, the genetic counselor reviews the status of screening for pancreatic cancer. Elizabeth expresses concern for pancreatic cancer given her uncle's diagnosis. The genetic counselor explains that currently there is no screening method that has proven effective for early detection of pancreatic cancer. Even so, for individuals at an increased risk for pancreatic cancer, some centers may offer investigational screening by imaging of the pancreas through endoscopic ultrasound and/or MRI, and possibly a specific tumor marker blood test. Elizabeth accepts information for some centers in the area who offer this investigational screening.

Like many patients, Elizabeth asks whether there are concerns of discrimination for people who test positive for a mutation. The genetic counselor reviews the current laws in place that have been developed to prevent genetic discrimination or using genetic information against an individual. The current federal law, Genetic Information Nondiscrimination Act (GINA), was passed in 2008 and offers protections in the areas of health insurance and employment discrimination. Health insurers may not use genetic information to make eligibility, coverage, underwriting, or premium-setting decisions. Employers may not use genetic information in employment decisions such as hiring, firing, promotions, and pay. The Genetic Information Nondiscrimination Act does not apply to the areas of life insurance, disability insurance, and long-term care insurance. The Genetic Information Nondiscrimination Act also does not apply to small employers (fewer than 15 employees) or to individuals who receive their insurance through the Federal Employees Health Benefits, the Veterans Health Administration, the U.S. Military, and the Indian Health Service. However, some of these other programs have their own established policies that prohibit different forms of genetic discrimination. Several states also have genetic discrimination laws in place, some of which offer greater protection than GINA and some of which offer less protection. If the state law is more protective than GINA, compliance with the more protective state law is required. In states previously with few or no protections, the federal regulations of GINA provide the baseline protections. (NHGRI, 2008).

As GINA does not provide protections related to life insurance, Elizabeth wants to review her current life insurance policy with her fiancé before deciding on genetic testing. The genetic counselor directs them to a few reliable online sources of information about genetic discrimination laws. Elizabeth calls the office back a couple of weeks later and decides to pursue genetic testing at that time. The genetic counselor schedules a follow-up appointment for Elizabeth to review her test results.

Elizabeth returns to the follow-up appointment with her fiancé. Her genetic test results are positive; she has the same mutation in the BRCA2 gene that was found in her mother. Elizabeth and her fiancé have discussed her options while waiting for her genetic test result and have decided not to pursue enhanced screening for breast cancer until after they have children, when she will consider a risk-reducing mastectomy and risk-reducing salpingo-oophorectomy.

Elizabeth's fiancé asks if there is a way to know if their future children also will have this BRCA2 gene mutation. The genetic counselor explains that the risk for any of their children would be 50%. She explains that genetic testing in childhood would not be recommended since BRCA2 mutations are not known to increase risk for childhood cancers and would not alter the child's medical management. Additionally, testing for mutations in the BRCA1 or BRCA2 genes is a personal decision, and testing of a child takes away his or her ability to make an informed and autonomous decision about genetic testing. The counselor also discusses reproductive genetic testing considerations. She explains that there is genetic testing that can be done during pregnancy for genetic conditions in the fetus, but that generally it is not useful or recommended in this situation unless the couple is considering termination of pregnancy. The counselor makes them aware of the option of in-vitro fertilization (IVF) with preimplantation genetic diagnosis (PGD), a procedure that would allow for BRCA2 genetic testing in the embryos before implantation of the embryos. The genetic counselor also discusses the rare instance in which a child may inherit two BRCA2 gene mutations (one from each parent), causing Fanconi anemia which is associated with childhood risks for bone marrow failure, different types of cancer, and sometimes physical differences. Elizabeth's fiancé states that he may consider his own BRCA2 gene testing to determine whether there is an increased risk of having a child with Fanconi anemia. The genetic counselor offers a referral to the reproductive genetics group to discuss these options in more detail, which Elizabeth and her fiancé accept.

Vignette #3: Woman with Prior Breast Cancer Diagnosis is Seen for Updated Genetic Testing (prior BRCA1/2 testing negative) and Tests Positive for Mutation in non-BRCA Breast Cancer Gene that Confers Moderate Breast Cancer Risk

Jean is a 63-year-old female with a past history of an invasive ductal carcinoma of the left breast at age 55. She underwent a lumpectomy, chemotherapy, and radiation therapy. She had her ovaries and uterus removed in her 40s due to ovarian cysts and endometriosis. Jean has one daughter and one son who are both in their late 30s. She previously saw a genetic counselor at the time of her breast cancer diagnosis. She had an additional family history of breast cancer in her mother, who was diagnosed at age 45, and in her maternal first cousin, who was diagnosed at age 50. At that time, she opted to have testing for BRCA1 and BRCA2 gene mutations and was negative. Jean has heard from a friend that there are new breast cancer genes that can be tested, and her friend encourages her to make another genetic counseling appointment.

The genetic counselor starts by updating Jean's family history. Jean's mother now is deceased, but there are no other major updates to Jean's family history. Jean admits she is a little confused about why she might need additional genetic testing since she already went through her breast cancer treatment. The genetic counselor reviews Jean's previous negative genetic testing which included the BRCA1 and the BRCA2 genes. The genetic counselor explains that Jean does not need to have the BRCA1 or BRCA2 gene test repeated, but that other genes more recently have been associated with an increased risk for breast cancer in some families. Some examples are the Partner and localizer of BRCA2 (PALB2), checkpoint kinase 2 (CHEK2) and ataxia telangiectasia mutated (ATM) genes. The genetic counselor explains that now it is possible to test for these genes together as part of a breast cancer gene panel or larger gene panel, which analyzes genes associated with breast cancer but also several other cancer types. These multi-gene panels may be appropriate for individuals who have had negative genetic testing previously, but a hereditary cause still is possible based on the personal or family history.

The genetic counselor reviews the benefits, risks, and limitations of testing for additional genes related to an increased risk for breast cancer. The counselor explains that while these genes increase a female's risk of developing breast cancer in her lifetime, the risk for most of the genes is lower than what has been observed in women who have mutations in the BRCA1 or BRCA2 genes. For that reason, they are sometimes referred to as "moderate risk" genes. The counselor reviews that the NCCN screening recommendations for women with mutations in CHEK2 and ATM include annual mammogram and breast MRI starting at age 40. The recommendations for women with mutations in the PALB2 gene include annual mammogram and breast MRI starting at age 30, with consideration of risk-reducing mastectomy based on family history. Jean asks the genetic counselor if there are any other cancers associated with mutations in these genes. The genetic counselor explains that some of the genes have been associated with increased risk for other types of cancers (such as ovarian cancer and pancreatic cancer with PALB2 mutations). However, for some of these genes, there may be limited or inconclusive evidence, and the exact risks may be unknown.

Jean decides to pursue the updated genetic testing panel. She comes to her follow-up appointment to receive her test results alone. Jean has a commonly observed mutation in the CHEK2 gene, which is written as '1100delC'. The genetic counselor reviews that this CHEK2 mutation has been found to confer an approximate 28% to 37% lifetime risk of developing a breast cancer (NCCN, 2017). Therefore, it is expected that this mutation played a significant role in the development of her breast cancer. It also indicates that Jean may have an increased risk for a second primary breast cancer; however, there still is not a lot of data on the specific risk. It was discussed that, in addition to her annual mammograms, she may wish to consider screening breast MRIs. Although there is no data on the benefit of risk-reducing mastectomy in women with CHEK2 mutations, some women may consider this based on family history (NCCN, 2017). In addition to increased risk for female breast cancer, mutations in the CHEK2 gene are associated with an elevated risk for male breast cancer and colorectal cancer (Meijers-Heijboer, 2002, and Xiang, 2011). The NCCN guidelines regarding CHEK2 mutations state that an individual without a history of colorectal cancer and with no family history of colorectal cancer, such as Jean, should have a colonoscopy every five years, beginning at the age of 40. Several studies discuss risk for other types of cancers related to CHEK2 gene mutations; however, the evidence is inconclusive and there are no current recommendations. Jean has never had a screening colonoscopy and decides to contact her primary care physician to get a referral as soon as possible. She also plans to discuss breast cancer screening with her breast surgeon and states that she may be interested in adding breast MRIs.

Jean asks the genetic counselor if her children should be tested. The genetic counselor reviews that because mutations in the CHEK2 gene are inherited in an autosomal dominant pattern, there is a 50% chance that each of her children have the same mutation in the CHEK2 gene. The counselor also discusses that testing will inform her children of their risk to develop the CHEK2-associated cancers and, therefore, help determine the type and age for appropriate screening.

Vignette #4: Woman with Prior Breast Cancer Tests Positive for Mutation in Unexpected Gene (e.g., postmeiotic segregation Increased, S.cerevisiae 2 (PMS2) Gene that is Associated with Lynch syndrome)

Victoria is a 45-year-old female with a history of a ductal carcinoma in-situ (DCIS) of one breast at age 43. Victoria opted to undergo a double mastectomy following her diagnosis. She has one healthy 23-year-old daughter. Victoria was previously seen by a genetic counselor following her breast cancer treatment to consider genetic testing. At that time, Victoria opted to have BRCA1 and BRCA2 mutation testing. She had negative genetic test results. Victoria's daughter recently saw a new primary care provider who asked her questions about her family history. Victoria's daughter now is more interested in learning about her own risk to develop breast cancer and encourages her mother to consider additional genetic testing.

Victoria meets with the same genetic counselor from two years ago who reviews and updates her family history. Victoria has a small family. She is an only child and her only uncle passed away at a young age. There is no family history of cancer. The genetic counselor reviews information about additional breast cancer genes and the availability of pursuing a breast cancer panel that will test these genes. She also discusses a larger, multi-gene cancer panel, which includes the genes associated with higher risk for breast cancer, but also genes associated with other types of hereditary cancer such as colorectal, endometrial, ovarian, and gastric cancer. Although there is a higher chance of identifying a gene variant of uncertain clinical significance or receiving an unexpected result when performing a larger, multi-gene panel, Victoria does not consider this to be a major drawback.

Victoria returns to the appointment with her daughter to receive her test results. To their surprise, she is found to have a mutation in the PMS2 gene. This is not a gene that has been customarily associated with hereditary breast cancer. Rather, it is one of the genes that can cause the hereditary cancer syndrome known as Lynch syndrome, which also is referred to as hereditary non-polyposis colorectal cancer. Mutations in the PMS2 gene increase risk primarily for colorectal and endometrial cancers; however, there also are believed to be some increased risks for ovarian, gastric, small bowel, brain, kidney, and ureter cancers. The genetic counselor explains to Victoria that there is emerging evidence to suggest that mutations in the PMS2 gene are more common in the general population than once thought, and there may be an associated increased risk for breast cancer in individuals with PMS2 gene mutations (Espenschied, 2017, and Win, 2017). Because Victoria's family is small and there is no family history of Lynch syndrome-associated cancers, it is difficult to know exactly what Victoria's risk is to develop these other cancer types such as colorectal and endometrial cancer. She is provided with a general estimation of PMS2-associated cancer risks and advised that she should follow the recommended screening and medical management guidelines for such. Specifically, the counselor reviews the current NCCN recommendations, which include an annual or biannual colonoscopy starting at age 20 to 25 years of age and consideration of risk-reducing hysterectomy and salpingo-oophorectomy.

Because currently there is no concrete evidence that breast cancer risk is increased in females with PMS2 gene mutations, the genetic counselor explains to Victoria's daughter that genetic testing would not change her screening recommendations for breast cancer at this time. Even if Victoria's daughter is negative for the PMS2 gene mutation found in her mother, she still will be considered to be at a higher risk for breast cancer based on her family history and should follow appropriate screening guidelines. Genetic testing for Victoria's daughter would be recommended, however, to determine her risk for developing established Lynch syndrome-associated cancers. Victoria's daughter decides to think about this information a little further and schedules a follow-up appointment for genetic counseling and testing in several months.

**Vignette #5: Woman with Breast Cancer who has
Negative Genetic Testing Result**

Abigail is a 50-year-old woman with a recent diagnosis of a ductal carcinoma in-situ (DCIS) of the right breast. She presents to the genetic counselor to discuss genetic testing for surgical decision-making. Abigail has no children and her ovaries and uterus are intact. The genetic counselor reviews her family history, which includes a mother who was diagnosed with ovarian cancer at age 55 and a maternal aunt who was diagnosed with breast cancer at age 60. Abigail's mother and maternal aunt are both still living and have never had genetic testing.

The genetic counselor reviews the purpose of genetic testing for surgical decision-making. The counselor discusses the benefits and limitations of BRCA1 and BRCA2 gene testing and multi-gene panel testing. The counselor explains that ovarian cancer can be due to mutations in genes such as BRCA1 and BRCA2 as well as other genes such as the Lynch syndrome-associated genes. Abigail is concerned about her risk for ovarian cancer and elects to proceed with a multi-gene cancer panel that will analyze all of these genes.

Abigail returns to her follow-up appointment with a friend to review her test results. Her results are negative; there were no mutations identified in any of the genes analyzed on the multi-gene panel. Abigail is shocked but relieved. The counselor explains that this negative result significantly reduces the likelihood that she has a hereditary form of breast cancer. A negative result cannot completely rule out the possibility of hereditary risk since there are some mutations that may not be detected. Abigail is informed that, most likely, her breast cancer is a sporadic occurrence or is multifactorial in nature, due to a combination of causes such as environmental factors and other types of genetic changes.

She has decided already that if her genetic test results are negative, indicating lower risk for a second primary breast cancer in the future, she will proceed with a lumpectomy rather than bilateral mastectomy. Abigail then expresses relief that she is now not at an increased risk for ovarian cancer and will not have to worry about this. The genetic counselor reminds Abigail that even though she was not found to have a mutation in any of the genes on the panel that are associated with ovarian cancer, she still is considered to be at increased risk based on her family history of ovarian cancer. The genetic counselor explains to Abigail that it is possible that her mother has a mutation in a gene associated with higher risk for ovarian cancer and that Abigail did not inherit this gene mutation. In order to better assess Abigail's risk for ovarian cancer, the genetic counselor recommends that Abigail discuss genetic testing with her mother. If Abigail's mother is found to have a mutation in a gene associated with higher risk for ovarian cancer, and Abigail does not have the same mutation, her risk for ovarian cancer will be significantly reduced. If Abigail's mother has negative genetic testing, in which case the cause of her ovarian cancer remains unknown, Abigail's risk for ovarian cancer will be considered to be significantly higher than the general population risk. This is based on data showing that women who have a first-degree relative with ovarian cancer have an approximate 3.1 times higher risk of developing ovarian cancer than the general population (Stratton, 1998). Abigail is encouraged to discuss ovarian screening and risk-reducing options with her gynecologist. Abigail believes her mother will be interested in genetic testing and decides to discuss this option with her.

SUMMARY

As illustrated in these examples, each individual who decides to undergo genetic risk assessment is unique. Factors that may affect decision-making include age, gender, education, cultural beliefs, religious beliefs, and lifetime experiences, including whether they have experienced a cancer diagnosis themselves or have been involved with a family member's diagnosis. Individuals also have different levels of anxiety, worry, and concern. In addition to the wide range among individuals who explore and undergo genetic testing, there also is a wide range of logistical differences in how this might be facilitated. Geographically, there are some regions in the country where there are many healthcare providers available who can facilitate this process of cancer risk assessment and counseling. In other areas, there may be no providers available, in which case tele-counseling by phone or video with a genetic counselor at a remote medical center, a genetic counseling service company, genetic testing laboratory, or health insurance company may be available. Cancer risk assessment and counseling also is provided by different types of healthcare providers. Although genetic testing traditionally has been facilitated by genetic counselors and geneticists and continues to be, it now is becoming more common for other types of healthcare providers to facilitate this. For example, many surgeons, oncologists, and oncology nurses now provide these services. This is often influenced by geographic location and the specific processes and referral patterns at individual medical offices and medical centers. Regardless of where and with whom the cancer risk assessment takes place, both pre-test counseling and post-test counseling should occur, as previously described.

For individuals who are interested in having a cancer risk assessment and genetic testing, the best way to initiate this is by discussing it with their personal physician(s) such as a primary care physician, nurse practitioner, gynecologist, surgeon, or oncologist. These care providers may have a referral system in place in which they easily refer patients to a local genetic counseling service. In some other situations, they may provide these services in their own offices. If they are not familiar with the genetic counseling services that are available in the area, patients can work to identify genetic counselors on their own. The main resource is the website of the National Society of Genetic Counselors (NSGC), available at http://www.nsgc.org/, which includes a "Find a Genetic Counselor" function. Another option is contacting the local hospital or medical center to determine if they have a genetics program that offers genetic testing. This information also may be accessible on their websites.

The study of breast cancer genetics is a fascinating and quickly evolving field and one that has an important impact on the individual and family. We expect that our understanding of breast cancer genetics and hereditary risk factors will continue to grow. This will likely lead to better characterization of the cancer risks associated with BRCA1 and BRCA2 gene mutations, better characterization of the cancer risks associated with other cancer susceptibility genes and different types of genetic changes and alterations, identification of new genes, development of more effective cancer therapies (particularly as it may relate to an individual's inherited gene mutation or to mutations within the tumor), and development of more effective cancer screening and prevention tools. This highlights the importance for genetics providers to keep up to date with the latest information on breast cancer genetics and for patients to keep in regular communication with their genetics provider and other healthcare providers. As our understanding of breast cancer genetics continues to develop, so does our ability to provide the most accurate risk assessment.

REFERENCES

1. Daly MB, Pilarski R, Berry M, Buys SS, Farmer M, Friedman S, Garber JE, Kauff ND, Khan S, Klein C, Kohlmann W, Kurian A, Litton JK, Madlensky L, Merajver SD, Offit K, Pal T, Reiser G, Shannon KM, Swisher E, Vinayak S, Voian NC, Weitzel JN, Wick MJ, Wiesner GL, Dwyer M, and Darlow S (2017). NCCN Guidelines Insights: Genetic/ Familial High-Risk Assessment: Breast and Ovarian, Version 2.2017. Journal of the National Comprehensive Cancer Network, 15(1):9-20.

2. Espenschied CR, LaDuca H, Li S, McFarland R, Gau CL, AND Hampel H (2017). Multigene panel testing provides a new perspective on lynch syndrome. Journal of Clinical Oncology, 35(22):2568-2575.

3. GINA federal law - https://seer.cancer.gov/statfacts/html/ovary.html

4. Hurst JH (2014). Pioneering geneticist Mary-Claire King receives the 2014 Lasker~Koshland Special Achievement Award in Medical Science. Journal of Clinical Investigation, 124(10):4148-4151.

5. King MC, Wieand S, Hale K, Lee M, Walsh T, Owens K, Tait J, Ford L, Dunn BK, Costantino J, Wickerham L, Wolmark N, and Fisher B (2001). Tamoxifen and breast cancer incidence among women with inherited mutations in BRCA1 and BRCA2: National Surgical Adjuvant Breast and Bowel Project (NSABP-P1) Breast Cancer Prevention Trial. JAMA, 286(18):2251–2256.

6. Mavaddat N, Peock S, Frost D, Ellis S, Platte R, Fineberg E, Evans DG, Izatt L, Eeles RA, Adlard J, Davidson R, Eccles D, Cole T, Cook J, Brewer C, Tischkowitz M, Douglas F, Hodgson S, Walker L, Porteous ME, Morrison PJ, Side LE, Kennedy MJ, Houghton C, Donaldson A, Rogers MT, Dorkins H, Miedzybrodzka Z, Gregory H, Eason J, Barwell J, McCann E, Murray A, Antoniou AC, and Easton DF (2013). Cancer risks for BRCA1 and BRCA2 mutation carriers: Results from prospective analysis of EMBRACE. Journal of the National Cancer Institute, 105(11):812–822.

7. Meijers-Heijboer H, van den Ouweland A, Klijn J, Wasielewski M, de Snoo A, Oldenburg R, Hollestelle A, Houben M, Crepin E, van Veghel-Plandsoen M, Elstrodt F, van Duijn C, Bartels C, Meijers C, Schutte M, McGuffog L, Thompson D, Easton D, Sodha N, Seal S, Barfoot R, Mangion J, Chang-Claude J, Eccles D, Eeles R, Evans DG, Houlston R, Murday V, Narod S, Peretz T, Peto J, Phelan C, Zhang HX, Szabo C, Devilee P, Goldgar D, Futreal PA, Nathanson KL, Weber B, Rahman N, and Stratton MR (2002). CHEK2-Breast Cancer Consortium. Low-penetrance susceptibility to breast cancer due to CHEK2(*)1100delC in noncarriers of BRCA1 or BRCA2 mutations. Nature Genetics, 31(1):55-59.

8. National Human Genome Research Institute: https://www.genome.gov/27568492/the-genetic-information-nondiscrimination-act-of-2008/

9. NIH SEER (general population breast cancer risk) https://seer.cancer.gov/statfacts/html/breast.html

10. NIH SEER (general population ovarian cancer risk) https://seer.cancer.gov/statfacts/html/ovary.html

11. Petrucelli N, Daly MB, and Pal T. BRCA1- and BRCA2-Associated Hereditary Breast and Ovarian Cancer. 1998 Sep 4 [Updated 2016 Dec 15]. In: Pagon RA, Adam MP, Ardinger HH, et al., editors. GeneReviews® [Internet]. Seattle (WA): University of Washington, Seattle; 1993-2017. Available from: https://www.ncbi.nlm.nih.gov/books/NBK1247/

12. Rebbeck TR, Lynch HT, Neuhausen SL, Narod SA, van't Veer L, Garber JE, Evans G, Isaacs C, Daly MB, Matloff E, Olopade OI, and Weber BL (2002). New England Journal of Medicine, 346(21):1616-22.

13. Stratton JF, Pharoah P, Smith SK, Easton D, and Ponder BA (1998). A systematic review

and meta-analysis of family history and risk of ovarian cancer. British Journal of Obstetrics and Gynaecology, 105(5):493-499.

14. Win AK, Jenkins MA, Dowty JG, Antoniou AC, Lee A, Giles GG, Buchanan DD, Clendenning M, Rosty C, Ahnen DJ, Thibodeau SN, Casey G, Gallinger S, Le Marchand L, Haile RW, Potter JD, Zheng Y, Lindor NM, Newcomb PA, Hopper JL, and MacInnis RJ (2017). Prevalence and penetrance of major genes and polygenes for colorectal cancer. Cancer Epidemiology, Biomarkers and Prevention, 26(3):404-412.

15. Xiang HP, Geng XP, Ge WW, and Li H (2011). Meta-analysis of CHEK2 1100delC variant and colorectal cancer susceptibility. European Journal of Cancer, 47(17):2546-2551.

A GYNECOLOGIST REVIEWS ESTROGEN'S RELATIONSHIP TO BREAST CANCER

James R. Woods, Jr., M.D., Elizabeth D. Warner, M.D., and
Adrienne D. Bonham, M.D., M.S.

The story of estrogen's relationship to breast cancer is complex. For many, the issue may seem straightforward. Estrogen causes breast cancer. Yet, if one examines the history of this supposed cause-effect relationship over time, many questions arise. Long before estrogen was discovered, when did ovarian function first become linked with breast cancer? And when did estrogen first become associated with ovarian function? Why was estrogen at one time successfully used to treat breast cancer? Why then did the Women's Health Initiative determine that hormone therapy was detrimental to women? What is the evidence that estrogen stimulates breast cancer cells under one circumstance and kills breast cancer cells at other times?

These are the questions often addressed in a gynecology office as breast cancer survivors seek care for menopause. These same questions are the source of confusion for many cancer survivors.

How prevalent is this healthcare issue? It seems that everyone either knows someone with breast cancer or has a personal or family experience with it. It is projected that in 2018, 266,120 new cases of invasive breast cancer and 63,960 cases of breast carcinoma *in situ* will be diagnosed, with 40,920 women dying of this disease (breastcancer.org).

This chapter is but a brief overview of a much more exhaustive story expanded upon by such authors as Rossouw (2002), Osborne (2005), Jordan (2011), Obiorah (2013), and Morch (2017).

DOES ESTROGEN CAUSE BREAST CANCER? A LITTLE HISTORY

As early as 1872, long before hormones were discovered, surgeons including Hegar (1872), Battey (1872), Nunn (1882) and others realized that oophorectomy had, for some reason, a beneficial effect on the course of the disease in certain women with breast cancer (Love, 2002). In 1895, Beatson reported on three cases of women with breast cancer, one of whom underwent bilateral oophorectomy in addition to the administration of sheep thyroid extract as treatment for the disease. By 1900, several surgeons were applying this approach to treat breast cancer with some success. In fact, in 1900, Boyd summarized available data which indicated that one-third of patients with breast cancer benefit from ovarian removal (Obiorah, 2013). However, it was not until 1923 when Allen and Doisy, by first showing that estrogen cornified the vaginal epithelium of mice and that the removal of ovaries reversed this process, identified estrogen as the hormone that is lost when the ovaries are removed.

WHY THEN WOULD SCIENTISTS ADVOCATE FOR THE BENEFITS OF ESTROGEN?

Even as studies of eliminating estrogen to reduce recurrence of breast cancer were ongoing, others were focusing their research on the benefits of estrogen for women in menopause. This concept was advanced publically in 1968 by Dr. Robert A. Wilson, a New York City gynecologist, in his book Feminine Forever (1968). He wrote, "the often-severe suffering of my menopausal patients made me regard menopause as a serious medical condition endangering the health and happiness of any woman..." Drawing from his experience with over 5,000 patients, he observed that, "In the vast majority of cases, the distressing bodily changes following menopause are reversible through estrogen treatment." The reactions of many feminists were robust and negative as they advocated for menopause as a natural part of life, not a disease, and, thus, required no "treatment."

At the same time, other researchers were examining the positive effects of estrogen upon cardiovascular health, supported by early studies in the monkey which showed that estrogen could inhibit the progression of postmenopausal atherosclerosis (Clarkson, 1996, and Ravas, 2002). Others were addressing the adverse relationship of menopause to bone health due to the loss of estrogen (Albright, 1941, and Lindsay, 1980).

DID THE WOMEN'S HEALTH INITIATIVE CLARIFY ESTROGEN'S RISK/BENEFIT?

The Women's Health Initiative (WHI) was begun in 1991, prompted by Dr. Bernadine Healy of NIH (National Institutes of Health) and funded by $725 million, to determine if hormone therapy (HT) in menopausal women would reduce coronary artery disease and osteoporosis (Women's Health Initiative Study Group, 1998). The study included 27,500 women, of whom 8,102 were randomized to placebo, and 8,506 to daily HT (known as Prempro®), which consisted of conjugated equine estrogen (CEE), 0.625 mg plus medroxyprogesterone acetate (MPA), 2.5 mg. For those women who had had a prior hysterectomy, 10,892 study participants were randomized to receive either estrogen therapy (ET), which consisted of CEE, 0.625 mg (Premarin®) alone, or placebo. The average age of WHI women at the start of the study was 63 years, with only 3.5% in the 50 to 54 age range. This would become an issue in later analyses of the results of the study.

The combined HT arm of the study was stopped after 5.2 years when it was noted that there was an increase in coronary heart disease (relative risk [RR] 1.24), as well as an increased risk of venous thrombosis and stroke among women who had taken HT. The item that caught the media attention, however, was an increased risk of breast cancer (RR 1.24) in this group. Causation was suggested by the fact that, after cessation of the study, there was a reduction in breast cancer among the remaining study participants. The beneficial aspects of HT were not widely publicized. Women who took HT were noted to have a decrease in the risk of endometrial cancer, osteoporotic fracture, and colorectal cancer.

In the original *Journal of the American Medical Association* report from 2002 (Rossouw, 2002), the authors wrote:

"Absolute excess risk per 10,000 years attributable to estrogen plus progestin were 7 more CHD (coronary heart disease) events, 8 more strokes, 8 more PEs (pulmonary emboli), and 8 more invasive breast cancers, while absolute risk reductions per 10,000 person-years were 6 fewer colorectal cancers and 5 fewer hip fractures. The absolute excess risk of events included in the global index was 19 per 10,000 person-years."

The remarkable (and not widely publicized) finding of this study was that after 6.8 years, the women who were given only CEE (0.625 mg/d) had a trend toward a decrease in coronary artery events with the best response for those 50 to 59 years (Anderson, 2004). While there was a 39% increase in stroke, there was a 30% reduction in bone fractures. Not only was there no increase in the risk of breast cancer among women who took estrogen alone, there was a 23% reduction in invasive breast cancer cases (six versus 16/10,000 person-years), with the greatest reduction in those without a family history of breast cancer or significant benign breast disease. Furthermore, if a woman did get breast cancer on estrogen, the mortality from breast cancer was reduced when compared to women who developed breast cancer while receiving a placebo (26 versus 33/10,000 person-years).

WHY WOULD HT HAVE A DIFFERENT EFFECT ON BREAST CANCER THAN ET ALONE?

High-dose estrogen has for decades been known to retard tumor growth. In 1935, Haddow, a microbiologist, observed that carcinogenic hydrocarbons retarded growth of malignant tumors (Haddow, 1935, 1974). In 1944, Haddow conducted the first trial of 73 women with advanced cancer, 40 with metastatic breast cancer, who were given either stilbestrol, triphenychlorethylene, or triphenymethlyethylene. Patients given stilbestrol or triphenylethylene showed signs of breast cancer reduction (Haddow, 1944).

The authors commented that in younger women, estrogen may accelerate mammary cancer. The beneficial responses of estrogens to reduce breast cancer are three times more frequent in women over the age of 60 than those under that age. Their therapeutic use, therefore, should be restricted to cases five years beyond menopause.

By the 1960s, high-dose stilbestrol was the treatment of choice for women with metastatic breast cancer, but the age of the patient made a difference in response. In one study of 407 women treated, 31% showed remission, but of 63 women in the first five years of menopause, only 9% showed remission, while those over five years into menopause had a 35% remission. Equally important, of those experiencing recurrence, a short treatment with estrogen produced a second, although shorter, remission (Stoll 1977).

BLOCKING ESTROGEN'S ACTIONS ON BREAST CANCER CELLS BY AN ANTI-ESTROGEN

So if estrogen can cause or stimulate breast cancer, can an antiestrogen or an estrogen blocker be able to prevent, inhibit, or kill breast cancer cells? Selective estrogen receptor modulators (SERMs) are chemically modified estrogens that, by targeting specific tissue estrogen receptors, block the estrogen response (Stevenson, 2007). Tamoxifen is a SERM that can block estrogen receptors in the breast. Tamoxifen trials of one, two, and five years in women with estrogen-positive breast cancer showed a decrease in recurrence of 21%, 29%, and 47%, respectively, independent of progesterone status, chemotherapy use, or age (Early Breast Cancer Trialists' Collaborative Group, 1998). Subsequently, a ten-year "Adjuvant Tamoxifen Longer Against Shorter Trial" (ATLAS) showed that ten years of tamoxifen treatment was better than five years (Davies, 2012). More significantly, there was a continued decrease in mortality after ten years of tamoxifen treatment was stopped, supporting a hypothesis put forth by Wolf in 1993 that a woman's own estrogen can destroy sensitive tamoxifen-resistant micrometastasis (Wolf, 1993).

WHAT IF CANCER CELLS BECOME RESISTANT TO ANTI-ESTROGEN TREATMENTS

The observation that breast cancer cells can become resistant to the estrogen-limiting actions of tamoxifen led to studies to explain this phenomenon. The ovariectomized MCF-7 athymic mice offered the best model for these studies since tumors mimicking human breast cancer can be generated in a laboratory. Following tamoxifen treatment, these tumors showed an initial regression that reversed with continued tamoxifen treatment. This observation suggested that breast cancer cells can develop tamoxifen drug resistance (Osborne, 1987). When tamoxifen-resistant tumors from MCF-7 athymic mice that had responded initially to tamoxifen were reimplanted into other MCF-7 athymic mice, the tumors continued to grow, even if then exposed to tamoxifen. Aromatase inhibiters, however, completely block any estrogen formation (estradiol, estrone) that would, under normal conditions, be formed in the body from androgen precursors. When a pure anti-estrogen was given to this mouse model, no further tumor growth was seen. Clinical support for a two-drug therapy was provided, since five years of aromatase-inhibitor therapy had proved valuable as an extended adjuvant treatment for postmenopausal women following five years of tamoxifen therapy (Goss, 2003). These observations led to the conclusion that if tamoxifen offers its effects primarily as a first-line treatment, it should be limited to only a few years, followed by a pure anti-estrogen of the aromatase-inhibitor family (Mouridsen, 2009, and Burstein, 2010).

In a subsequent study, MCF-7 mice tamoxifen-treated tumors were transplanted into other athymic mice that had been pretreated with tamoxifen for five years before the transplant. After the transplant, when tamoxifen was stopped, tumors continued to regress, suggesting that the animal's own estrogens now were destroying any remaining breast cancer cells (Wolf, 1993).

WHY WOULD ESTROGEN KILL CANCER CELLS?

Apoptosis or programmed cell death is a genetically engineered process that, when activated, leads to cell death. This process differs from necrosis in which the cell appears to break apart and induce an inflammatory response in nearby tissues. In apoptosis, the cells shrink and condense with the cytoskeleton collapsing and the DNA breaking up. These cell surface changes induce phagocytosis by other cells (Murray, 2012). Apoptosis involves proteolytic enzymes called caspases that, when activated, result in cell death. This process is regulated tightly by such inhibitors as Bcl-2.

It now is recognized that estrogen induces stress within the endoplasmic reticulum and induces an inflammatory response, thus resulting in cellular apoptosis. Severe stress has been shown to override the blocking actions of Bcl (Ariazi 2011). Tamoxifen promotes apoptosis by activating the death receptor, Fas, and suppressing certain anti-apoptotic transcription factors (Osipo, 2003).

The process of apoptosis is influenced by the cellular levels of glutathione (GSH) produced through the actions of two enzymes, GSH synthetase, and GSH peroxidase 2. Resistance to chemotherapy-induced apoptosis is linked to over-expression of Bcl-2, which elevates glutathione (GSH) levels and blocks a critical step in apoptosis, (the weakening of the outer membrane of mitochondria), leading to release of cytochrome C and caspase 9. Once GSH is depleted, apoptosis is restored as shown in a study where MCF-7:2A cells were exposed to estradiol plus a GSH inhibitor, and the frequency of apoptosis was increased (Lewis-Wambi, 2008, 2009).

It is premised that women treated with CEE immediately after onset of menopause may experience sustained growth of nascent estrogen-receptor positive tumor cells. Beyond five years after menopause, estrogen exposure in these estrogen-depleted breast cells may produce apoptosis (Jordan, 2003, 2011, and Lewis, 2005).

The paradox that a woman's own estrogen may destroy pre-sensitized breast cancer cells after five years of tamoxifen treatment offers the possibility of step-wise management of breast cancer. Furthermore, tumors that regrow after estrogen-induced apoptosis generate cancer cells with the original cancer phenotype and, thus, would be sensitive to antitumor actions of anti-estrogen treatment (Yao, 2000).

SO WHY DID HT BUT NOT ET ALONE INCREASE BREAST CANCER IN WOMEN IN THE WHI? WHAT ABOUT HORMONAL CONTRACEPTION?

Considerable debate targets the question whether micronized (natural) progesterone or synthetic progestins can increase the risk of breast cancer alone or when combined with estrogen, prescribed either as contraceptive pills or menopausal HT. While the role of natural progesterone on the uterus during the menstrual cycle is well known, progesterone's actions on the breast are less well appreciated. During the reproductive years, the proliferative phase leading up to ovulation is dominated by estrogen. In the luteal phase, progesterone dominates.

The human **breast epithelium** is a branching ductal system composed of an inner layer of polarized luminal epithelial cells and an outer layer of myoepithelial cells that terminate in distally located terminal duct lobular units. During the luteal phase, breast epithelium proliferates, peaking nine to ten days after ovulation, particularly in the terminal duct lobular units, which is the site where most breast cancers develop (Ferguson, 1981, and Russo, 1990). It is during the luteal phase that breast cells normally undergo apoptosis and sloughing of breast epithelium occurs, peaking just before menses begins (Longacre, 1986). It is debated, however, whether the changes in breast epithelium are from progesterone or a delay in effect of estrogen. One could speculate that the increase in breast cancer with continuous combined estrogen and progestin (rather than natural progesterone) may be the result of sustained estrogen/progestin use, which prevents shedding of the breast epithelium. One may also speculate as to whether these effects would be seen with the use of natural progesterone as opposed to other types of progestins such as medroxyprogesterone acetate used in the WHI study.

In a population-based, case-controlled study of former and current oral contraceptive users age 35 to 64, 4,575 women with breast cancer and 4,682 controls were interviewed. No significant increase in breast cancer was found, even when length of use, race, or family history was accounted for (Marchbanks, 2002).

Other, more recent reviews have challenged that observation. From an extensive review by Campagnoli (2005), as well as more recent reports (Samson, 2016, and Morch, 2017), synthetic progestins, when added to estrogen, are linked to an increased risk of breast cancer. This conclusion is drawn from numerous studies demonstrating an inability to slough mammary epithelium when the progestin is withdrawn as occurs in a normal cycle, as well as decreased insulin sensitivity, increased insulin-like growth factor-1 (with its mitogenic anti-apoptotic effects on breast cancer cells), and decreased sex-binding globulin, which leads to elevated free testosterone levels. All of these conditions are associated with an increased breast cancer risk.

More significantly, two studies have failed to demonstrate an increase in the risk of breast cancer with natural progesterone use. In one, 3,175 menopausal women were followed for a mean of 8.9 years; 53% were on HT consisting of transdermal estrogen with either a natural progesterone or progestins other than MPA, the derivative used in the WHI (de Lignieres, 2002). No increase in breast cancer was detected. In a larger study of 54,548 postmenopausal women who entered the program without any hormone treatments for at least one year (mean age 52.8 years), the addition of a synthetic progestin with an estrogen significantly increased the risk for breast cancer, even in as short an exposure period as two years, while use of estrogen and natural progesterone produced no increased risk (Fournier, 2005).

CONCLUSION

The histories of estrogen and breast cancer are complicated, dating to the 1800s. While the public attitude often is reduced to "estrogen produces breast cancer," scientists challenge this simplistic conclusion. Initial observations drawn from the WHI resulted not only in a dramatic reduction in prescriptions for HT but also a dilemma for gynecologists managing women suffering from menopausal symptoms. In prescribing HT or ET, a physician must take into account the timing of initiation, route of delivery, choice of progesterone, length of treatment, side effects, and risks in view of patient's medical/family history along with the patient's desires and reasons for treatment. Prescribing hormonal contraception (whatever the route) with the small but present increased risk of breast cancer also requires a similar study of risks versus benefits. Today, a more balanced approach is available, yet the responsibility still rests with the gynecologist to present the facts to our patients whom we are trying to help through these chapters of their lives.

REFERENCES

1. Albright F, Smith PH, and Richardson AM (1941). Postmenopausal osteoporosis-its clinical features. JAMA, 116:2465-2473.

2. Anderson GL, Limacher MC, Assaf AR, Bassford T, Beresford SA, Black H, Bonds D, Brunner R, Brzyski R, Caan B, Chlebowski R, and Curb D (2004). Effects of conjugated equine estrogen in postmenopausal women with hysterectomy: The Women's Health Initiative randomized controlled trial. JAMA, 291:1701-1712.

3. Ariazi EA, Cunliffe HE, Lewis-Wambi JS, Slifker MJ, Willis AL, Ramos P, Tapia C, Kim HR, Yerrum S, Sharma CGN, Nicolas E, Balagurunathan Y, Ross EA, and Jordan VC (2011). Estrogen induces apoptosis in estrogen deprivation-resistant breast cancer through stress responses as identified by global gene expression across time. Proceedings of the National Academy of Sciences of the United States of America, 108(47):18879-18886.

4. Burstein HJ, Prestrud AA, Seidenfeld J, Anderson H, Buchholz TA, Davidson NE, Gelmon KE, Giordano SH, Hudis CA, Malin J, Mamounas EP, Rowden D, Solky AJ, Sowers MR, Stearns V, Winer EP, Somerfield MR, and Griggs JJ (2010). Clinical practice guideline: update on adjuvant endocrine therapy for women with hormone receptor-positive breast cancer. Journal of Clinical Oncology, 28(23):3784-3796.

5. Campagnoli C, Clavel-Chapelon F, Kaake R, Peris C, and Berrino F (2005). Progestins and progesterone in hormone replacement therapy and the risk of breast cancer. Journal of Steroid Biochemistry and Molecular Biology, 96(2):95-108.

6. Clarkson TB, Anthony MS, and Klein KP (1996). Hormone replacement therapy and coronary artery atherosclerosis: The monkey model. British Journal of Obstetrics and Gynaecology, 103; Suppl 13; 53-57.

7. Davies C, Pan H, Godwin J, Gray R, Arriagada R, Raina V, Abraham M, Alencar VHM, Baran A, Bonfill X, Bradbury J, Clarke M, Collins R, Davis SR, Delmestri A, Forbes JF, Haddad P, Hou M, and Inbar M (2012). Long-term effects of continuous adjuvant tamoxifen to 10 years versus stopping at 5 years after diagnosis of oestrogen receptor-positive breast cancer; ATLAS, a randomized trial. Lancet, 381(9869):805-816.

8. De Lignieres B (2002). Effects of progestogens on the postmenopausal breast. Climacteric, 5(3):229-235.

9. Early Breast Cancer Trialists' Collaborative Group (1998). Tamoxifen for early breast cancer: An overview of the randomized trials. Lancet, 351(9114):1451-1467.

10. Ferguson DJ and Anderson TJ (1981). Morphological evaluation of cell turnover in relation to the menstrual cycle in the "resting" human breast. British Journal of Cancer, 44(2):177-181.

11. Fournier A, Berrino F, Riboli E, Avenel V, and Clavel-Chapelon F (2005). Breast cancer risk in relation to different types of hormone replacement therapy in the E3N-EPIC cohort. International Journal of Cancer, 114(3):448-454.

12. Goss PE, Ingle JN, Martino S, Robert NJ, Muss HB, Piccart MJ, Castiglione M, Tu D, Shepherd LE, Pritchard KI, Livingston RB, Davidson NE, Norton L, Perez EA, Abrams JS, Therasse P, Palmer MJ, and Pater JL (2003). A randomized trial of letrozole in postmenoausal women. New England Journal of Medicine, 349(19):1793-1802.

13. Haddow A (1974). An autobiographical essay. Cancer Research, 34(12):3159-3164.

14. Haddow A (1935). Influence of certain polycyclic hydrocarbins on the growth of the Jensen Rat sarcoma. Nature, 136: 68-869.

15. Haddow A, Watkinson JM, and Paterson E (1944). Influence of synthetic oestrogens upon advanced malignant disease. BMJ, 2:393-398.

16. Jordan VC (2003). Tamoxifen: A most unlikely pioneering medicine. Nat Rev Drug Discovery (2003) 2; 205-213.

17. Jordan VC and Ford LG (2011). Paradoxical clinical effect of estrogen on breast cancer risk: A "new" biology of estrogen-induced apoptosis. Cancer Prevention Research, 4(5):633-637.

18. Lewis JS, Meeke K, Osipo C, Ross EA, Kidawi N, Li T, Bell E, Chandel NS, and Jordan VC (2005). Intrinsic apoptosis in breast cancer cells resistant to estrogen deprivation. Journal of the National Cancer Institute, 97(23):1746-1759.

19. Lewis-Wambi J, Kim H, Wambi C, Patel R, Pyle JR, Klein-Szanto AJ, and Jordan VC (2008). Buthionine sulfoximine sensitizes anti-hormone-resistant human breast cancer cells to estrogen-induced apoptosis. Breast Cancer Research, 10(6): R104.

20. Lewis-Wambi J and Jordan VC (2009). Estrogen regulation of apoptosis: How can one hormone stimulate and inhibit? Breast Cancer Research, 11:206.

21. Lindsay R, Hart DM, Forrest C, and Baird C (1980). Prevention of spinal osteoporosis in oophorectomized women. Lancet, 2:1151-1154.

22. Longacre TA and Bartow SA (1986). A correlative morphologic study of human breast and endometrium in the menstrual cycle. American Journal of Surgical Pathology, 10(6):382-393.

23. Love RR and Philips J (2002), Oophorectomy for breast cancer; history revisited. Journal of the National Cancer Institute, 94:1434-1435.

24. Marchanks PA, McDonald JA, Wilson HG, Folger SG, Mandel MG, Daling JR, Bernstein L, Malone KE, Ursin G, Strom BL, Norman SA, Wingo PA, Burkman RT, Berlin JA, Simon MS, Spirtas R, and Weiss LK (2002). Oral contraceptives and the risk of breast cancer. New England Journal of Medicine, 346; 2025-2032.

25. Morch LS, Skovlund CW, Hannaford PC, Iversen L, Fielding S, and Lidegaard O (2017). Contemporary hormone contraception and the risk of breast cancer. New England Journal of Medicine, 377:2228-2239.

26. Mouridsen H, Giobbie-Hurder A, Goldhirsch A, Thürlimann B, Paridaens R, Smith I, Mauriac L, Forbes J, Price KN, Regan MM, Gelber RD, and Coates AS (2009). Letrozole therapy alone or in sequence with tamoxifen in women with breast cancer. New England Journal of Medicine, 361:766-776.

27. Murray RK, Jacom M, and Varghese J (2012). Cancer: An overview (Chapter 55). In: RK Murray, DA Bender, KM Botham, PJ Kennelly, VW Rodwell, Weil PA (Eds.). Harper's Illustrated Biochemistry, (Ed. 29). New York: Lange McGraw Hill, 696-717.

28. Obiorah I and Jordan VC (2013). Scientific rationale for postmenopause delay in the use of conjugated equine estrogens among postmenopausal women that causes reduction in breast cancer incidence and mortality. Menopause, 20:372-382.

29. Orkun T, Bradshaw K, and Bruce C (2012). Management of vulvovaginal atrophy-related sexual dysfunction in postmenopausal women. Menopause, 19:109-117.

30. Osborne CK (1993). Mechanisms for tamoxifen resistance in breast cancer: Possible role of tamoxifen metabolism. Journal of Steroid Biochemistry and Molecular Biology, 47:83-89.

31. Osborne CK and Schiff R (2005). Estrogen-receptor biology; continuing progress and therapeutic implications. Journal of Clinical Oncology, 23(8):1616-1622.

32. Osborne CK, Coronado LB, and Robinson JP (1987). Human breast cancer in the athymic nude mouse: Cytostatic effects of long-term antiestrogen therapy. European Journal of Cancer and Clinical Oncology, 23(8):1189-1196.

33. Osipo C, Gajdos C, Liu H, Chen B, and Jordan VC (2003). Paradoxical action of fulvestrant in estradiol-induced regression of tamoxifen-stimulated breast cancer. Journal of the National Cancer Institute, 95(21):1597-1608.

34. Ravas RH (2002). Animal models of the cardiovascular effects of exogenous hormones. American Journal of Cardiology, 90(1A):22F-25F.

35. Russo J, Gusterson BA, Rogers AE, Russo IH, Wellings SR, and van Zwieten MJ (1990). Comparative study of human and rat mammary tumorigenesis. Laboratory Investigation, 62(3):244-278.

36. Rossouw JE, Anderson GL, Prentice RL, LaCroix AZ, Kooperberg C, Stefanick ML, Jackson RD, Beresford SA, Howard BV, Johnson KC, Kotchen JM, and Ockene J. Writing Group for the Women's Health Initiative Investigators (2002). Risks and benefits of estrogen plus progestin in healthy postmenopausal women: Principal results from the Women's Health Initiative Investigators. JAMA, 288(3):321-333.

37. Samson M, Porter N, Orekoya O, Hebert JR, Adams SA, Bennet CL, and Steck SE (2016). Progestin and breast cancer risk: A systematic review. Breast Cancer Research and Treatment, 155(1):3-12.

38. Stevenson S and Thornton J (2007). Effect of estrogens on skin aging and the potential role of SERMS. Clinical Interventions in Aging, 2(3):283-297.

39. Stoll B (1977). Palliation by castration or by hormone administration. In: BA Stoll, (Ed.). Breast Cancer Management Early and Late. London: William Heinemann Medical Books Ltd, 133-146.

40. The Women's Health Initiative Study Group (1998). Design of the Women's Health Initiative clinical trial and observational study. Controlled Clinical Trials, 19(1): 61-109.

41. Wilson RA (1968). Feminine Forever. New York: Pocket Books.

42. Wolf D and Jordan VC (1993). A laboratory model to explain the survival advantage observed in patients after taking adjuvant Tamoxifen therapy. Recent Results in Cancer Research, 127:23-33.

43. Yao K, Lee ES, Bentrem DJ, England G, Schafer JI, O'Regan RM, and Jordan VC (2000). Antitumor action of physiological estradiol on tamoxifen-stimulated breast tumors grown in athymic mice. Clinical Cancer Research, 6(5):2028-2036.

TRIPLE-NEGATIVE BREAST CANCER

Thomas D. Rodgers, Jr., M.D. and Alissa J. Huston, M.D.

During their lifetime, nearly one in eight women will sit in oncology offices across the United States (U.S.) discussing their new diagnosis of breast cancer (Bauer, 2007). In these visits, many words and phrases will be mentioned: surgery, chemotherapy, estrogen receptor status, and Her2 protein; however, for a portion of these women, two words will linger, "triple-negative." So often in medicine, negative results are mentioned in a favorable light, such as "your biopsy was negative." Unfortunately, it is not likely that these words will be received in the same manner. Due to the absence of estrogen and progesterone receptor positivity along with lack of HER2 overexpression, these women will learn that triple-negative breast cancer is a more aggressive disease with a higher chance of relapse. For many, the full definition and history, as well as the significant current research, may be lost through a web of details. In this chapter, we will explore this diagnosis and provide a framework for healthcare workers, patients, and their patients' families to understand better and confront a diagnosis of triple-negative breast cancer.

We will start this chapter with a case, that of Ms. G., a 35-year-old African-American woman who has three young children and leads a busy life. After feeling a left breast mass, she went to see her primary care doctor and was sent for an ultrasound and mammogram. An abnormal area was discovered and biopsied. Sitting across from her new oncologist, she is told she has triple-negative breast cancer, limited to her left breast, and that she will require chemotherapy, surgery, and likely radiation. She is shocked, given her young age, and she asks several questions. Is this a different form of breast cancer than others? How did this happen? Is this more aggressive than other forms of breast cancer? Can this be treated? To help better understand triple-negative breast cancer and ultimately answer these questions, we will follow the case of Ms. G. through the many intricacies of the diagnosis.

IS THIS A DIFFERENT FORM OF BREAST CANCER?

The simple answer to this questions is "yes." However, this answer hardly encapsulates how we define breast cancer. Triple-negative breast cancer is less a specific diagnosis and more a description of a tumor that lacks three commonly identified breast tumor markers: the estrogen receptor (ER), progesterone receptor (PR), and HER2-neu protein overexpression. Thus, breast cancer generally has been categorized based on these markers as a hormone-responsive disease (ER and/or PR positive), HER2-positive disease, or triple-negative disease (the absence of ER, PR, and HER2 overexpression). These have become our framework for diagnosing breast cancer type, and they largely define treatment paradigms. In addition, they provide prognostic information for the individual and her family.

Best characterized by Jensen in 1971, the estrogen receptor has proven to be the most important indicator of response to endocrine therapy and is a useful tool to help predict disease course (Jensen, 1971). The estrogen receptor sits on the tumor cell wall, and breast cancers with this receptor can respond to circulating hormones. When estrogen binds to this receptor, a cascade of messages are sent to increase cellular proliferation, ultimately leading to tumor growth. For this reason, it was hypothesized that blocking this receptor could help treat breast cancer.

In the 1970s, this hypothesis was proven correct, and tamoxifen was developed (Jordan, 1976). Tamoxifen works by allowing for the modulation of this signaling pathway by binding to the estrogen receptor, leading to a decreased response to circulating hormones (Powles, 1989). Hormonal manipulation with tamoxifen and aromatase inhibitors has since become the backbone of treatment for those with estrogen or progesterone receptor-positive disease (Fisher, 1998). Additional therapies are necessary if a patient has HER2 positive disease. HER2 is a protein that, when overexpressed, promotes cancer growth. In 1998, the FDA approved the monoclonal antibody trastuzumab (Herceptin®) to treat HER2-positive disease (Paik, 2008), and additional targeted therapies have been approved since that time. While many therapies exist for HER2- and estrogen-positive disease, no approved specific cellular target has been identified in triple-negative disease. For this reason, chemotherapy has been the standard treatment.

Although triple-negative breast cancer differs from hormone-responsive disease and HER2-positive disease, it does not represent a homogeneous group of tumors. Research at the molecular level has led to the determination of six subtypes of triple-negative breast cancer, including basal-like 1, basal-like 2, immunomodulatory, mesenchymal-like, mesenchymal stem-like, and luminal androgen-receptor subtype. These subtypes are centered around different gene expression, receptor positivity, and unique histology (Lehmann, 2011, and Hubalek, 2017). For example, those with the luminal androgen receptor subtype have overexpression of the androgen receptor, and those with immunomodulatory have distinct changes in the tumor immune microenvironment. Although there are no FDA-approved therapies currently that target each subtype, the discovery of the subtypes provides hope for future research and therapeutic targets.

HOW DID THIS HAPPEN?

As with almost every cancer, there is no single answer. Cancer development is a complex and varied path that often includes a balance between inherent predisposition, sporadic mutations, and environmental factors. In triple-negative disease, as of yet, there has not been one specific mutation or commonly identified modifiable risk factor leading to its development. Instead, there are certain prevailing trends in its diagnosis. Triple-negative breast cancer accounts for approximately 15% of all newly diagnosed breast cancers across the U.S. When taking into account that nearly 250,000 women in the U.S. were estimated to have been diagnosed with breast cancer in 2017, about 38,000 of those women were told that their disease was triple-negative. These 38,000 women tend to have a few characteristics in common (DeSantis, 2017).

Unfortunately, as with our patient Ms. G., triple-negative breast cancer disproportionately affects the young and premenopausal population. In fact, approximately 60% of those with triple-negative breast cancer are diagnosed before the age of 60. Additionally, for reasons not yet known, African-American women are two to three times more likely than Caucasian women to have triple-negative disease. Taken another way, nearly 40% of premenopausal African-American women diagnosed with breast cancer will have triple-negative disease. This is compared to 15% in the same young Caucasian population (Carey, 2006). At 35 years of age, Ms. G.'s diagnosis is in line with current trends. Other trends have been noted in this population, including an increased prevalence of patients with a BRCA1 or BRCA2 mutation. These mutations most often are inherited and lead to an increased probability of developing breast cancer. While only 5% of patients with breast cancer have a BRCA mutation, 20% to 30% of patients with triple-negative breast cancer are thought to have a BRCA mutation (Malone, 2006, and Greenup, 2013).

IS THIS TYPE MORE AGGRESSIVE?

Unfortunately, the answer to this question is yes. Those with triple-negative breast cancer have worse outcomes when compared to hormone-responsive disease across all breast cancer stages. It is most notable, perhaps, in advanced or metastatic disease where five-year survival is more than 20% reduced in triple-negative disease as compared to those with hormone-responsive disease (Bauer, 2007). For these reasons, being given a diagnosis of triple-negative breast cancer can be devastating to a patient and her family. However, there is reason to be hopeful. This is because research is rapidly identifying more tailored chemotherapy regimens, which are finding success in the treatment of triple-negative breast cancer. Additionally, more personalized targets are being discovered, even in a group previously defined by its lack of common markers. Along with the different subtypes of triple-negative disease, there are varied response rates; some people respond well to treatment and have excellent long-term outcomes. Still, there are others with reduced response rates. Current research is underway to define this population and develop more personalized therapies.

CAN THIS BE TREATED?

Back to the case: Ms. G. has just discovered that she has triple-negative breast cancer and that it is more common in young African-American women than in young Caucasian women. She knows from having done research online that the disease is more aggressive and outcomes tend to be worse compared to other forms of breast cancer. When she asks, "Can this be treated?" The unequivocal answer is "yes."

Standard treatment varies depending on the specific stage of cancer, with definitive surgery either occurring before or after chemotherapy in nonmetastatic disease to long-term chemotherapy in stage IV disease. In both settings, the specifics of the chemotherapy along with research into directed therapies are driving a changing treatment paradigm.

TREATMENT IN TRIPLE-NEGATIVE BREAST CANCER

While a complete review of all treatment regimens is not possible in this chapter, following our patient Ms. G. through treatment allows for a glimpse into the options that exist within triple-negative breast cancer. She felt a left breast mass that prompted her to seek medical care through her primary care provider. She was sent quickly to have an ultrasound and mammogram performed, which demonstrated a sizeable, left-sided mass along with a suspicious enlarged axillary lymph node. After a biopsy of both, the breast mass and axillary lymph node demonstrated triple-negative invasive ductal carcinoma, and she was referred to a medical oncologist. There she was staged as having stage IIB breast cancer.

While treatment with chemotherapy often is reserved for large or high-risk tumors in hormone response disease, chemotherapy is recommended for even small tumors with triple-negative breast cancer. In fact, current National Comprehensive Cancer Network (NCCN) guidelines recommend chemotherapy for all patients with tumors greater than 1 cm and with the consideration of treatment in those with tumors greater than 5 mm. It also is agreed widely that any patient with lymph node-positive disease, regardless of the tumor size, should receive chemotherapy if she has triple-negative breast cancer (Costa, 2017). As Ms. G. had a tumor over 1 cm, it was recommended that she undergo systemic chemotherapy. If potentially resectable, chemotherapy can either be given before surgery (neoadjuvant) or after surgery (adjuvant setting). This decision often is driven by the patient's desire or ability to receive breast-conserving therapy. As she hoped to be able to undergo breast-conserving surgery, neoadjuvant chemotherapy was recommended.

In the neoadjuvant setting, chemotherapy is the mainstay treatment to shrink the tumor. Additionally, a tumor's response to therapy leading up to surgery has been shown to be predictive of patient outcome. Those without evidence of cancer on mastectomy samples after chemotherapy have significantly prolonged overall survival compared to those who have residual disease. For example, over 90% of patients who have a pathologic complete response (pCR) were alive at eight years in a recently completed study. Unfortunately, only 25% of patients with poor response rates were alive at eight years (Symmans, 2017). For this reason, treatment in the neoadjuvant setting has been directed at obtaining a complete response or lack of cancer on the final surgical specimen.

Common neoadjuvant treatments include chemotherapy combinations using a category of drugs called taxanes. For hormone-responsive disease, a common regimen could consist of docetaxel and cyclophosphamide or the more aggressive regimen of doxorubicin and cyclophosphamide. For triple-negative breast cancer, standard treatment has been to side with more aggressive therapy, thus favoring the combination of doxorubicin and cyclophosphamide followed by paclitaxel (Taxol®), often referred to as AC+T.

While this regimen in studies has led to improved response rates across many forms of cancer, the addition of another chemotherapy type in triple-negative breast cancer is being researched. Platinum-based agents such as carboplatin were first shown to have efficacy in patients with metastatic disease. Recent studies incorporating carboplatin into neoadjuvant treatment protocols have been shown to improve outcomes and increase the chance of a complete response to therapy. Pathologic complete response (pCR) has been considered a surrogate endpoint for overall survival in patients with triple-negative breast cancer. Therefore, many studies have been aimed at improving the outcome in the neoadjuvant setting. Two large Phase II Trials have studied the addition of carboplatin to Taxol® in the neoadjuvant setting—GeparSixto Trial and CALGB40603 (von Minckwitz, 2014, and Sikov, 2015). These studies both have demonstrated an improvement in the pCR rates with the addition of carboplatin, yet have been mixed in terms of event-free survival (EFS), although neither initially was designed or powered for this endpoint. GeparSixto has demonstrated an improvement in EFS, while this has not been shown for CALGB40603. That being said, this combination also has been shown to be more toxic with an increased chance of developing severe drops in blood counts and the need to reduce or discontinue additional doses. Previous studies have demonstrated this can occur in up to 40% to 50% of those receiving the additional chemotherapy. This continues to remain a very active area of research with current trials investigating the role of carboplatin as a single agent following neoadjuvant chemotherapy for those with residual disease (von Minckwitz, 2014).

Given the importance of a complete response, clinical trials have investigated the addition of adjuvant chemotherapy to improve outcomes for those patients unable to obtain a complete response. Unfortunately, this was the case for our patient Ms. G., as she had residual disease on her mastectomy biopsy. For this reason, adjuvant therapy was discussed and ultimately started. Adjuvant capecitabine was chosen based on the results of the Create-X trial. In this study, adjuvant capecitabine was studied in patients with residual cancer on mastectomy samples after neoadjuvant therapy. This study demonstrated a nearly 10% improvement in five-year overall survival with the addition of adjuvant capecitabine (Masuda, 2017). Apart from capecitabine, further trials are ongoing investigating the use of platinum-based agents in the adjuvant setting (NCT02488967 and NCT02445391).

NOVEL THERAPIES

It is hoped that in the future, the term triple-negative will become obsolete, as it is a term that reflects our ignorance of the disease. Future directions in the area of triple-negative breast cancer research are highly focused on identifying new targets for metastatic disease. Apart from unique chemotherapy regimens, areas of active research include identifying novel agents and regimens such as the use of cell cycle checkpoint inhibitors in the immunomodulatory subtype, antiandrogen therapy in luminal androgen receptor subtype, and the use of Poly (ADP-ribose) polymerase (PARP) inhibitors in those with BRCA mutations.

Briefly, in the immunomodulatory subtype, there is upregulation of many genes including signal transducers and activators of transcription (STAT) factors, leading to alterations in B and T-cell function in the tumor microenvironment. While only consisting of around 20% of diagnosed triple-negative breast cancer, it was hypothesized that this subtype might have improved responses with cell cycle checkpoint immunotherapy. The KEYNOTE-012 study confirmed this hypothesis as a subset of patients had a durable response (Nanda, 2016). Antiandrogen therapy is an additional area of investigation for those patients with luminal androgen-receptor positive breast cancer. In this subtype, androgen receptor positivity is nearly ten times higher than those with other subtypes. Several trials are ongoing with androgen receptor-blocking agents, including bicalutamide, enzalutamide, and abiraterone (Mina, 2017). Finally, those with BRCA mutations have been found to have improved response rates with the use of PARP inhibitors (Robson, 2017).

CONCLUSION

As we learn more about the diverse heterogeneity of triple-negative breast cancer, our hope is to improve upon standard chemotherapy by developing new regimens and identifying novel targets. In this way, it is conceivable that research may render the term triple-negative obsolete as we develop more personalized therapy across the variety of this diagnosis. While triple-negative breast cancer remains a challenging diagnosis, there are reasons to be hopeful. Although studies are ongoing, recent advances already have been included in clinical practice and have provided patient benefit. The case of Ms. G. provides an example of this benefit, as she completed additional adjuvant therapy with capecitabine to reduce her risk of cancer recurrence. In the future, we hope to extend such benefits to other women through ongoing research.

REFERENCES

1. Bauer KR, Brown M, Cress RD, Parise CA, and Caggiano V (2007). Descriptive analysis of estrogen receptor (ER)-negative, progesterone receptor (PR)-negative, and HER2-negative invasive breast cancer, the so-called triple-negative phenotype: A population-based study from the California Cancer Registry. Cancer, 109(9):1721-1728.

2. Carey LA, Perou CM, Livasy CA, Dressler LG, Cowan D, Conway K, Karaca G, Troester MA, Tse CK, Edmiston S, Deming SL, Geradts J, Cheang MC, Nielsen TO, Moorman PG, Earp HS, and Millikan RC (2006). Race, breast cancer subtypes, and survival in the Carolina Breast Cancer Study. JAMA, 295(21):2492-2502.

3. Costa RLB and Gradishar WJ (2017). Triple-negative breast cancer: Current practice and future directions. Journal of Oncology Practice, 13(5):301-303.

4. DeSantis CE, Ma J, Goding Sauer A, Newman LA, and Jemal A (2017). Breast cancer statistics, 2017, racial disparity in mortality by state. CA: A Cancer Journal for Clinicians, 67(6):439-448.

5. Fisher B, Costantino JP, Wickerham DL, Cecchini RS, Cronin WM, Robidoux A, Bevers TB, Kavanah MT, Atkins JN, Margolese RG, Runowicz CD, James JM, Ford LG, and Wolmark N (1998). Tamoxifen for prevention of breast cancer: Report of the National Surgical Adjuvant Breast and Bowel Project P-1 Study. Journal of the National Cancer Institute, 90(18):1371-1388.

6. Greenup R, Buchanan A, Lorizio W, Rhoads K, Chan S, Leedom T, King R, McLennan J, Crawford B, Kelly Marcom P, and Shelley Hwang E (2013). Prevalence of BRCA mutations among women with triple-negative breast cancer (TNBC) in a genetic counseling cohort. Annals of Surgical Oncology, 20(10):3254-3258.

7. Hubalek M, Czech T, and Müller H (2017). Biological subtypes of triple-negative breast cancer. Breast Care, 12(1):8-14.

8. Jensen EV, Block GE, Smith S, Kyser K, and DeSombre ER (1971). Estrogen receptors and breast cancer response to adrenalectomy. National Cancer Institute Monograph, 34:55-70.

9. Jordan VC (1976). Effect of tamoxifen (ICI 46,474) on initiation and growth of DMBA-induced rat mammary carcinomata. European Journal of Cancer (Oxford, England : 1990). 12(6):419-424.

10. Lehmann BD, Bauer JA, Chen X, Sanders ME, Chakravarthy AB, Shyr Y, and Pietenpol JA (2011). Identification of human triple-negative breast cancer subtypes and preclinical models for selection of targeted therapies. The Journal of Clinical Investigation, 121(7):2750-2767.

11. Malone KE, Daling JR, Doody DR, Hsu L, Bernstein L, Coates RJ, Marchbanks PA, Simon MS, McDonald JA, Norman SA, Strom BL, Burkman RT, Ursin G, Deapen D, Weiss LK, Folger S, Madeoy JJ, Friedrichsen DM, Suter NM, Humphrey MC, Spirtas R, and Ostrander EA (2006). Prevalence and predictors of BRCA1 and BRCA2 mutations in a population-based study of breast cancer in white and black American women ages 35 to 64 years. Cancer Research, 66(16):8297-8308.

12. Masuda N, Lee S-J, Ohtani S, Im Y-H, Lee E-S, Yokota I, Kuroi K, Im S-A, Park B-W, Kim S-B, Yanagita Y, Ohno S, Takao S, Aogi K, Iwata H, Jeong J, Kim A, Park K-H, Sasano H, Ohashi Y, and Toi M (2017). Adjuvant capecitabine for breast cancer after preoperative chemotherapy. New England Journal of Medicine, 376(22):2147-2159.

13. Mina A, Yoder R, and Sharma P (2017). Targeting the androgen receptor in triple-negative breast cancer: Current perspectives. OncoTargets and Therapy, 10:4675-85.

14. Nanda R, Chow LQ, Dees EC, Berger R, Gupta S, Geva R, Pusztai L, Pathiraja K, Aktan G, Cheng JD, Karantza V, and Buisseret L (2016). Pembrolizumab in patients with advanced triple-negative breast cancer: Phase Ib KEYNOTE-012 Study. Journal of Clinical Oncology, 34(21):2460-2467.

15. Paik S, Kim C, and Wolmark N (2008). HER2 status and benefit from adjuvant trastuzumab in breast cancer. New England Journal of Medicine, 358(13):1409-1411.

16. Powles TJ, Hardy JR, Ashley SE, Farrington GM, Cosgrove D, Davey JB, Dowsett M, McKinna JA, Nash AG, and Sinnett HD (1989). A pilot trial to evaluate the acute toxicity and feasibility of tamoxifen for prevention of breast cancer. British Journal of Cancer, 60(1):126-131.

17. Robson M, Im S-A, Senkus E, Xu B, Domchek SM, Masuda N, Delaloge S, Li W, Tung N, Armstrong A, Wu W, Goessl C, Runswick S, and Conte P (2017). Olaparib for Metastatic Breast Cancer in Patients with a Germline BRCA Mutation. New England Journal of Medicine, 377(6):523-533.

18. Sikov WM, Berry DA, Perou CM, Singh B, Cirrincione CT, Tolaney SM, Kuzma CS, Pluard TJ, Somlo G, Port ER, Golshan M, Bellon JR, Collyar D, Hahn OM, Carey LA, Hudis CA, and Winer EP (2015). Impact of the addition of carboplatin and/or bevacizumab to neoadjuvant once-per-week paclitaxel followed by dose-dense doxorubicin and cyclophosphamide on pathologic complete response rates in stage II to III triple-negative breast cancer: CALGB 40603 (Alliance). Journal of Clinical Oncology, 33(1):13-21.

19. Symmans WF, Wei C, Gould R, Yu X, Zhang Y, Liu M, Walls A, Bousamra A, Ramineni M, Sinn B, Hunt K, Buchholz TA, Valero V, Buzdar AU, Yang W, Brewster AM, Moulder S, Pusztai L, Hatzis C, and Hortobagyi GN (2017). Long-term prognostic risk after neoadjuvant chemotherapy associated with residual cancer burden and breast cancer subtype. Journal of Clinical Oncology: Official Journal of the American Society of Clinical Oncology, 35(10):1049-1060.

20. von Minckwitz G, Schneeweiss A, Loibl S, Salat C, Denkert C, Rezai M, Blohmer JU, Jackisch C, Paepke S, Gerber B, Zahm DM, Kümmel S, Eidtmann H, Klare P, Huober J, Costa S, Tesch H, Hanusch C, Hilfrich J, Khandan F, Fasching PA, Sinn BV, Engels K, Mehta K, Nekljudova V, and Untch M (2014). Neoadjuvant carboplatin in patients with triple-negative and HER2-positive early breast cancer (GeparSixto; GBG 66): A randomised phase 2 trial. The Lancet Oncology,15(7):747-756.

BREAST RECONSTRUCTION:
KNOWING THE OPTIONS

Ashley N. Amalfi, M.D. and Elaina Y. Chen, M.D.

INTRODUCTION

Breast reconstruction is one of the many facets of Breast Cancer care. The decisions that women face in choosing to pursue breast reconstruction often are the most personal. All women should be informed of their reconstruction options and offered a method that is safe and effective, and that allows them to feel beautiful, feminine, and comfortable with their body after breast cancer.

The decisions women need to make regarding reconstruction depend upon which type of oncologic surgery they pursue: partial or total mastectomy. For women having a partial mastectomy, modern techniques allow for the rearrangement of local tissue to create a breast with a pleasing contour and shape. If pursuing a total mastectomy, there are various options to reconstruct the entire breast using either a breast implant, autologous tissue from the patient's own body, or a combination of both. Some women may choose to have both breasts removed as a method of reducing their risk of breast cancer on the side that is not affected, but that decision could be made later. In certain circumstances, the oncologic surgeon also may offer a nipple-sparing mastectomy. When only one breast is operated on, women have options for various procedures on their healthy breast to help them achieve symmetry.

Many women express concerns regarding whether breast reconstruction is financially feasible. The Women's Health and Cancer Rights Act of 1998 (WHCRA) is a federal law that was passed to provide protections to patients who choose to have breast reconstruction following mastectomy (Centers for Medicare & Medicaid Services, 2017). This includes coverage for not only the primary reconstructive efforts but also any resulting complications and, oftentimes, subsequent procedures to achieve a satisfactory result. Despite this legislation still less than half of all women requiring mastectomy are offered or informed of breast reconstruction options. Fewer than one in five patients choose to undergo reconstruction. In response to this, the American Society of Plastic Surgeons (ASPS) worked with Congress to pass the Breast Cancer Patient Education Act of 2015, which required the Secretary of Health and Human Services to plan and implement an education campaign to inform breast cancer patients of the availability and coverage of breast reconstruction (H.R.2540 - Breast Cancer Patient Education Act of 2015). The goal is for all women to be educated and informed of their right to pursue breast reconstruction that is reimbursed by insurance. A breast oncology surgeon should provide basic information to patients about reconstruction and a referral to a plastic surgeon for further evaluation for patients who demonstrate interest in knowing more about their reconstructive options.

TIMING OF RECONSTRUCTION

Breast reconstruction can be performed either immediately following mastectomy or delayed for some time after mastectomy. The advantages of immediate reconstruction include combining two procedures in a single anesthetic. Also, psychologically, many women find it more acceptable to wake up with a breast in the early stages of reconstruction rather than to a flat chest. In immediate reconstruction, the breast cancer surgeon also can preserve more of the breast skin that will be used by the plastic surgeon for reconstruction.

Delayed reconstruction may be the ideal choice for women who are smokers or for patients who cannot withstand the long duration of general anesthesia necessary for a combined procedure. Some women may require immediate adjuvant oncologic treatment and it would not be safe to pursue reconstruction and possibly delay their other therapies. Similarly, some women do not elect to have reconstruction at the time of their mastectomy but may choose reconstruction in the future. The amount of time that has passed between mastectomy and reconstruction generally does not limit a patient's choices.

CANDIDACY FOR RECONSTRUCTION

Being a good candidate for reconstruction is multifactorial. The plastic surgeon must first and foremost consider the safety of reconstruction as it relates to each patient's overall health, cancer treatment regimen, and expected complication profile.

Each woman's medical history is paramount when considering her candidacy for breast reconstruction. Patients who are otherwise healthy are safe candidates for surgery. Patients who have major heart disease, respiratory problems, kidney failure, neurologic dysfunction, and bleeding or clotting tendencies need evaluation by their plastic surgeon and other medical providers to assess their individual risk. Some women with very large tumors or metastatic disease may require chemotherapy or other cancer therapy prior to surgery. These decisions regarding candidacy for reconstruction in such patients are made by the entire breast cancer treatment team, taking into account multiple factors that make each patient unique.

Oncologic Surgery

There are a variety of mastectomy types that will affect the type of reconstruction a woman pursues. The original surgical treatment for breast cancer was the radical mastectomy, which removed not only the breast tissue but all of the breast skin, pectoralis muscles, and lymph nodes in the axilla. This was a very debilitating surgery that is performed extremely rarely today. The modified radical mastectomy is a modern variation of the radical mastectomy that spares the pectoralis muscles and some breast skin, but still removes the axillary lymph nodes in entirety. A total mastectomy consists of the removal of breast tissue and just enough breast skin to be able to close the skin together, leaving the chest wall flat. This can be combined with a sentinel lymph node biopsy. When a woman chooses immediate reconstruction, a skin sparing mastectomy is performed to preserve the breast skin to be used for the reconstructed breast. Most recently, nipple-sparing procedures have proven to be oncologically safe for many women. The criteria for nipple-sparing mastectomy continue to evolve, and women who desire this option should discuss the safety with their oncologic surgeon. For women who desire reconstruction with a nipple-sparing approach, the ideal candidate is small breasted with appropriately positioned nipples and minimal ptosis, or drooping, of the breast. Nipple-sparing mastectomy has the highest reported patient satisfaction rates and best reported aesthetic outcomes after breast reconstruction, likely because the breast skin envelope is completely preserved, and the native nipple areolar complex is difficult to replicate in reconstruction.

Smoking

Nicotine, most commonly in the form of cigarette smoking or vaping, is one of the biggest risk factors for complications related to breast reconstruction surgery. The use of nicotine compromises blood flow in capillaries, the smallest blood vessels in the body. In mastectomy, this is important especially because the arteries carrying blood to the skin are typically removed with the breast tissue, leaving behind skin that must survive on blood flow through a small capillary network. Nicotine use can lead to devastating consequences, including wound healing problems, infection, and ultimately failure of reconstruction. The plastic surgeon may choose to delay any reconstruction until the patient has abstained from nicotine products for at least two months before and after surgery to prevent these disastrous complications.

Radiation

Radiation is an important adjunct to breast cancer treatment that may influence the reconstructive plan. The changes to the tissue and skin of the chest following radiation exposure have profound implications on breast reconstruction techniques and timing. Studies have shown that radiation exposure either before or after reconstruction with an implant leads to higher rates of infection, implant loss, and wound healing complications (Krueger, 2001, and Sbitany, 2014). Patients with radiation also have reported lower satisfaction with their breasts and outcomes, with lower rates of psychosocial, sexual, and physical well-being compared with non-irradiated patients (Albornoz, 2014). For these reasons, autologous reconstruction using a woman's own tissue often is a better choice in this setting.

Obesity

Obesity, defined as a body mass index greater than 30 kg/m^2, is a growing epidemic worldwide, affecting at least one-third of adults in the United States (U.S.). Obesity itself is not necessarily a contraindication to reconstruction, but progressively higher BMIs have been associated with higher rates of complications, including wound healing problems, pneumonia, pulmonary embolism, postoperative renal insufficiency, urinary tract infection, stroke, myocardial infarction, symptomatic deep venous thrombosis, sepsis, infections, graft and prosthesis loss, and unplanned return to the operating room (Fischer, 2013). Breast implants do not come in sizes large enough for some people, due to higher complication rates with extremely large implants. Obesity also can make autologous reconstruction more difficult technically and a less ideal option in some women.

Age

Reconstruction is performed less frequently in women of advanced age, but age alone is not a contraindication to reconstruction. There is, however, a higher likelihood that an elderly patient may have multiple health problems that can affect her candidacy for certain types of reconstructions.

Hypercoagulable States

A plastic surgeon will evaluate a patient's personal and family history of blood clots, multiple miscarriages, or a known blood clotting disorder. Medical conditions such as factor V Leiden deficiency, protein S or C deficiency, lupus anticoagulant, and others may be a contraindication to autologous free flap reconstruction due to the risk of anastomotic thrombosis or clotting of the blood vessels that are re-connected.

TYPES OF RECONSTRUCTION

Breast reconstruction falls into three general categories: implant based, autologous, or a combination of these. Implant-based reconstruction is the most frequently used method of reconstruction, with 70% to 80% of women choosing this option. This operation has the benefit of shorter operative times but usually requires multiple surgeries to reach the final result. Autologous reconstruction uses a patient's own tissue from another part of her body to recreate a breast, is technically more demanding, and requires longer operative times. This method of reconstruction is completed in one surgery, but many women choose to undergo minor secondary revisions to perfect their result. If a larger breast is desired, a patient's own tissue may sometimes be combined with a breast implant to give a volume that fits the patient's body and desires.

Anecdotal experience has shown that most women are quite satisfied with their reconstructed breasts. Ultimately, the type of reconstruction that is right for each patient is determined by her candidacy for certain procedures, her preferences and desires, and her surgeon's ability to perform those procedures.

IMPLANT-BASED RECONSTRUCTION

Implant reconstructions typically are performed in two stages. The first stage involves the placement of a breast tissue expander, which is designed to stretch the chest skin and tissue until the desired final breast size is achieved. The tissue expander can be placed during the same procedure as the mastectomy. During surgery, it is filled slightly with saline, or sterile salt water, to create the initial mound of the breast. After an initial recovery period of one to two weeks, it is then injected with more saline weekly to slowly stretch the remaining tissues to support a permanent breast implant. New tissue expanders are available now that use a built-in carbon dioxide cartridge to fill the expander with gas without the use of needles and saline in the office. The filling process is controlled by a remote, which allows the patient to perform her own expansion safely and more gradually from the comfort of her own home (www.airxpanders.com). Whether the expander is filled with water or air, the final size of the reconstruction is determined by both the patient and her surgeon based on the patient's preference, anatomy, and other individual characteristics.

The tissue expander can be placed in a variety of positions within the chest. Traditionally, it is placed in a total submuscular plane below the pectoralis muscle and the serratus muscle of the lateral chest. An alternative technique that has gained popularity involves using the pectoralis muscle for upper implant coverage and acellular dermal matrix, or cadaver dermis, to support and cover the remainder of the expander. The acellular dermal matrix acts like an internal brassiere that gives contour to the lower pole of the breast, creating a more natural ptotic shape that mimics the native breast contour. This product also allows the surgeon to use more saline to fill the expander at the time of placement, creating a more fully expanded breast at the time of the initial surgery (Sbitany, 2009). Over time, acellular dermal matrix becomes incorporated into the patient's body. The major disadvantage of acellular dermal matrix is that its use may increase the rate of seroma, or fluid buildup around the breast implant, which may lead to more infections (Jordan, 2016). Some plastic surgeons prefer to wrap the entire breast implant in acellular dermal matrix and place it on top of the muscle in a prepectoral plane. The advantage of this is less postoperative pain and a more comfortable expansion process with a similar safety profile (Sbitany, 2017).

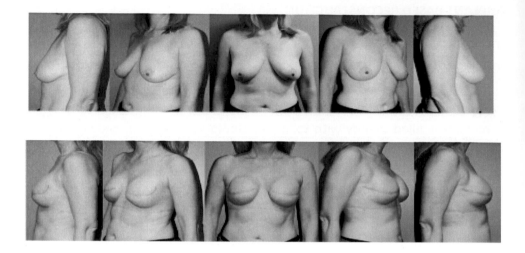

Figure 1. Patient with Tissue Expanders in Place

When the patient has been expanded to her desired size, she is then ready for her second stage surgery. This may occur a few months following the initial tissue expander placement, or it may be delayed to accommodate chemotherapy and radiation therapy. During this second stage, the tissue expander is removed and replaced with a permanent breast implant. At this time, fat grafting also may be performed to achieve a more pleasing appearance of the breast. Fat grafting is described in more detail later in this chapter.

Occasionally, reconstruction can be performed in a single stage with a permanent implant placed at the initial surgery in a select group of patients. In many of these patients, revision surgeries still are necessary to achieve an optimal aesthetic result.

Implant Selection

All breast implants are composed of an outer silicone shell. This shell may be filled with either saline solution or silicone gel. Saline is 0.9% sodium chloride in water, which is the same solution that is often used for intravenous fluid therapy. Silicone is a synthetic gel filling that is more viscous than saline and feels more like natural tissue. Tissue expanders have a thicker silicone shell and are filled via a magnetic port with saline solution. There are a variety of sizes, shapes, and variations that surgeons can use based on patient anatomy and personal preference (Figure 2).

Breast implants were first approved for use through the United States Federal Drug Administration (FDA) in 1976. After almost two decades of use for both cosmetic and reconstructive procedures, concern emerged over a possible association between silicone implants and various systemic adverse effects such as the development of connective tissue diseases. The FDA issued a moratorium in 1992 on the use of silicone gel-filled implants for patients undergoing primary

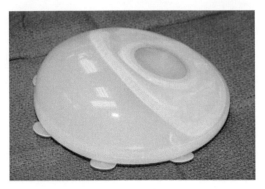

Figure 2. Tissue Expander Device

breast augmentation surgery, but still allowed their use for breast reconstruction patients and patients undergoing implant revision surgeries. Multiple studies were performed to evaluate the safety of silicone gel-filled implants and, in 2006, the moratorium was lifted when no correlation was found between the implants and associated systemic illness (USFDA, 2017a).

Silicone implants quickly regained their popularity in breast surgery and remain a safe and effective option for many women. These implants range from very liquid viscosity gels to more form-stable cohesive gels. The more liquid silicone gel is deformable and can change its shape based on body position, gravity, and external forces. Form-stable cohesive gel, or "gummy bear" gel, is less deformable, does not change its shape based on body position or gravity, and is resistant to external forces. The implant, when cut, resembles the inside of a gummy bear candy, hence its nickname (Figure 3).

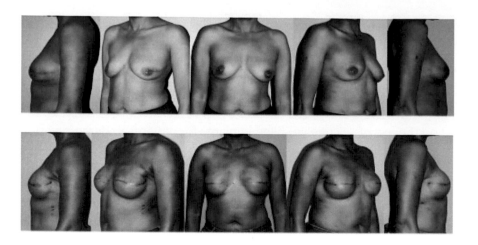

Figure 3. Patient Preoperatively and with Final Silicone Implant Reconstruction

Silicone often is chosen for its natural feel, which is especially important in the reconstructive population, as the implant is directly palpable beneath the skin following a mastectomy. As breast implants are man-made devices, rupture is a possible, albeit a rare outcome of the procedure. When a silicone implant has ruptured, it is not absorbed by the body, making it difficult for both the patient and plastic surgeon to detect. To this end, the FDA recommends magnetic resonance imaging (MRI) surveillance of silicone gel-filled implants three years after implant placement and then every other year thereafter (USFDA, 2017b).

Saline implants have remained an option in both cosmetic and reconstructive surgery. They offer the advantage of easy detection of rupture, as the saline is absorbed quickly by the body and immediately identified by the patient. Replacement of saline implants is a simple operation and offers patients peace of mind that a rupture will be both easily detected and straightforward to treat.

Breast implants come in a variety of shapes and sizes. They may be round or shaped. The shaped anatomic implant, also referred to as a teardrop implant, has a slimmer upper profile and more projection in the lower pole, making it appear similar to a natural breast. In contrast, a round implant has equal projection on all sides (Figure 4). However, gravity allows the lower viscosity gels to take a more anatomic shape when the patient sits up, creating a very natural look as well.

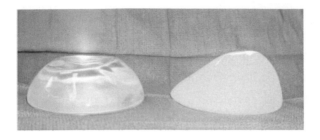

Figure 4. Round versus Shaped Implants

The outer shell of the implant may be smooth or textured. The smooth devices are designed to move around within their capsule in the body. Textured implants have a rough surface and grip the surrounding tissue much like Velcro®. This keeps the implant in an exact position. This is an optimal choice for a shaped implant, as the texturing keeps the teardrop implant from rotating and creating a distorted shape.

Breast Implant-Associated Anaplastic Large Cell Lymphoma

Breast implant-associated anaplastic large cell lymphoma (BIA-ALCL) is a rare form of lymphoma that has been diagnosed in the capsules surrounding breast implants. This rare non-Hodgkin's lymphoma is a cancer of T lymphocytes and may be related to chronic inflammation exacerbated by the texturing of breast implants. To date, 359 patients with BIA-ALCL have been reported to the FDA (USFDA, 2017c). Breast implant-associated anaplastic large cell lymphoma usually presents an average of seven years after implant placement with new and sudden swelling of one breast from fluid around the implant, pain, or a mass (Loch-Wilkinson, 2017). If suspected, a plastic surgeon will test the fluid or mass for cellular markers indicative of BIA-ALCL. When diagnosed, BIA-ALCL is highly treatable by removing the breast implant and the capsule that surrounds it. Occasionally, adjuvant chemotherapy is required. Death from BIA-ALCL is extremely rare.

AUTOLOGOUS RECONSTRUCTION

Autologous reconstruction involves using a patient's own tissue from another part of her body to reconstruct her breast. The benefits of this are that the reconstruction can be completed in a single surgical stage, and the final result is very natural in both appearance and feel. Autologous reconstruction is technically more demanding, and the operative times are much longer. As the breast is completed during the initial surgery, there are fewer postoperative visits, and there is no required secondary procedure. However, many women do choose to undergo minor revisionary procedures to optimize the breast contour with fat grafting, to further shape the breast, or to pursue nipple and areolar reconstruction.

In autologous reconstruction, skin, fat, and muscle may be borrowed from nearby or distant sites in the body. When using nearby tissue, or *regional* tissue, the artery supplying that tissue remains connected to the body, and is termed a *pedicled flap*, or *pedicled tissue transfer*. If the tissue borrowed is from a more distant location in the body, the artery supplying that tissue must be divided and then reconnected to another blood vessel in the chest to re-establish blood flow to the tissue, much like a transplant. This is termed a *free flap* or *free tissue transfer*.

REGIONAL TISSUE TRANSFER OPTIONS

Regional or pedicled flaps may be used to reconstruct the breast. The two most common pedicled flaps for breast reconstruction are the *latissimus dorsi (LD) muscle or myocutaneous flap,* and the *transverse rectus abdominis muscle or myocutaneous (TRAM) flap*. A muscle flap involves the transfer of muscle alone, whereas a myocutaneous flap includes the muscle and the overlying skin and fat.

Latissimus Dorsi Muscle or Myocutaneous Flap

The latissimus dorsi is a muscle found in the back that assists with shoulder motion. It is the largest muscle of the body, spanning the entire middle and lower back. It can be used in breast reconstruction with very little functional deficit, as the other local muscles help to stabilize and maintain shoulder function. The LD muscle is harvested with overlying fat and skin to create a breast mound. It remains attached to its blood supply, the thoracodorsal artery and vein, which is located in the axilla. It then is rotated from its position on the back, while maintaining its arterial connections, and placed in the front of the chest to reconstruct the breast. If a patient does not have enough fat or tissue on her back to make a large enough breast, an implant or tissue expander may be placed below the latissimus flap to create a larger breast. Fat grafting may be combined with the latissimus flap to increase volume as well (Figure 5). The scar created on the back is large; however, it does create a back lift effect and often improves the contour of the back and sides. The surgeon will often design the scar to be hidden underneath a standard brassiere.

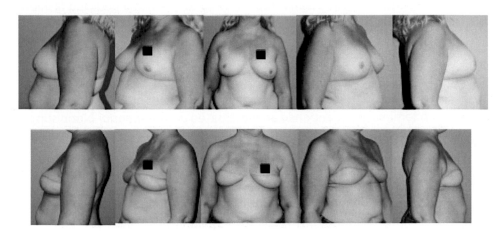

**Figure 5. Patient with Latissimus Dorsi Myocutaneous
Flap Reconstruction with Fat Grafting**

Transverse Rectus Abdominis Muscle or Myocutaneous Flap

The rectus abdominis muscle is found in the abdomen and assists with flexing the torso. Combined with the other abdominal wall muscles, it is important for maintaining posture of the torso and spine and can be seen in very muscular individuals as a "six pack." It can be used in breast reconstruction as a regional flap, transferring the entire muscle from the abdomen up to the chest while keeping it attached to its superior blood supply, the superior epigastric artery and vein. This flap is a good choice for a unilateral reconstruction. It should not be used for bilateral reconstruction, as moving both muscles would greatly destabilize the torso. This flap removes the lower abdominal skin and fat, akin to a tummy tuck or abdominoplasty, and moves this up to the chest to create a breast mound. Many patients favor an abdominal donor site as with the TRAM flap, because it also serves to recontour and tighten the lower abdomen. Women may experience weakening of the abdominal wall following this procedure, in which a hernia or bulge can develop. This is seen more commonly in women who are less physically fit or overweight. The pivot point of the flap from the abdomen to the chest can also sometimes be bulky.

FREE TISSUE TRANSFER OPTIONS

Free tissue transfer involves the division of a tissue's blood supply from the donor site and reconnection to the recipient blood vessels in the chest. This technique is necessary when the donor tissue is too far away to reach in a pedicled fashion. There are several options of donor sites throughout the body that can be used to reconstruct the breast with a free tissue transfer.

Abdominally Based Free Tissue Transfer

The rectus abdominis flap mentioned above is based on the *superior* blood supply when used as a regional option. The use of this muscle as a free tissue transfer is based on the more dominant *inferior* blood supply, the inferior epigastric artery, and vein. Variable amounts of the muscle may be harvested with the overlying fat and skin, called a *free muscle-sparing transverse rectus abdominis myocutaneous (free msTRAM) flap*. In a more technically demanding procedure, the fat and skin can be isolated on a single branch, or *perforator*, from the deep inferior epigastric artery, termed a *deep inferior epigastric artery perforator (DIEP) flap*. This approach spares the harvest of the muscle entirely, making the flap comprised of fat and skin only.

Occasionally, a more superficial blood vessel can be found to be predominantly supplying the abdominal fat and skin, called the *superficial inferior epigastric artery (SIEA) flap*. This flap has no risk of hernia formation, as the muscle itself is not violated; however, it has less consistent anatomy than the free TRAM or DIEP flaps and is less commonly available for use. Ultimately, the type of abdominally based flap used is dependent on several variables, including patient anatomy and the surgeon's preference and specific skill set.

An abdominal donor site is an enticing option to many patients, and the volume obtained usually is adequate to provide a pleasing final result in a single stage. As with the pedicled TRAM flap, the free flaps from the abdomen also provide an abdominoplasty type of result to the donor site. The major disadvantage of these flaps involves weakening of the abdominal wall and hernia or bulge at the donor site. It is important to note that the abdomen can be used to reconstruct either one or both breasts in a single stage, but once it is used for unilateral reconstruction, it cannot be used again at a future date for contralateral reconstruction.

Transverse Upper Gracilis Flap

The transverse upper gracilis (TUG) flap, also known as the inner thigh flap, uses skin, fat, and the gracilis muscle from the inner thigh to reconstruct the breast. The gracilis muscle serves a minor role in bringing the thighs together. The blood vessels that supply this flap are the medial femoral circumflex artery and vein. This method is useful for patients who do not have an adequate abdominal or back donor site. As with the other flaps discussed, there are minimal functional deficits following harvest of the gracilis muscle. The unique crescent shape of this tissue allows it to be sculpted into a circular shape with some conical projection to mimic a natural breast. The donor site has the advantage of being recontoured like a medial thighplasty, leaving a pleasing resultant thigh donor site. The major difference between the TUG and abdominally based reconstructions is that the TUG must use a smaller piece of tissue, which may be of insufficient volume in larger breasted patients.

Superior Gluteal Artery Perforator Flap

The superior gluteal artery perforator (SGAP) flap includes only skin and fat harvested in the region of the superior buttocks, based on a perforating blood vessel from the superior gluteal artery and vein. Since this is a perforator flap that does not require muscle harvest, there is no functional deficit from its usage. This flap is considered when the abdominal donor site is not available and the TUG flap is too small. The volume obtained from this flap is dependent on each patient's individual anatomy, but generally, it is smaller than an abdominal flap and larger than an inner thigh flap. The dissection for this flap can be technically challenging for an inexperienced surgeon, and the resultant donor site scar is large and traverses horizontally across the upper buttocks. However, this incision usually is designed to be hidden underneath the waistband of standard undergarments.

FAT GRAFTING

Fat grafting involves the collection of fat from unwanted areas such as the abdomen, flanks, and hips using liposuction, and then re-injecting the fat into the chest for primary

103

breast reconstruction, or to add volume to another reconstructive modality. Fat grafts are unlike flaps, because they do not have their own blood supply. Instead, they rely on the vascularized tissue into which they are injected to provide the necessary nutrients for them to survive. Fat grafts must be meticulously processed after harvesting. Newer technology available to surgeons now allows ease of fat procurement for the surgeon, enabling larger volumes of fat to be injected and for better graft survival within the recipient tissue (Figure 6). Volume retention with these newer techniques is about 60% with skillful and meticulous processes, compared to about 30% with older techniques.

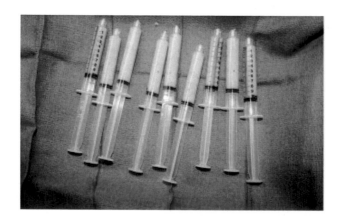

Figure 6. Fat Grafting

Fat grafting can be used as an adjunct procedure in both implant-based and autologous reconstructions. For implant-based reconstruction, fat grafting typically is performed at or after the second stage, when the tissue expander is exchanged for a permanent implant. Fat may be injected to fill any contour abnormalities of the mastectomy flaps, and to improve the shape of the breast and its harmony with the chest. In an autologous reconstruction, fat grafting may be used in a similar fashion to improve contour and to augment volume by direct injection into the flap.

NIPPLE AND AREOLA RECONSTRUCTION

The final stage of reconstruction is the creation of a new nipple-areolar complex (NAC). This last stage is optional, but many women find that once it has been completed, they are able to truly and finally accept a reconstructed breast as part of their own bodies. There are a variety of different ways to reconstruct a nipple, using local tissues for nipple creation only or with full thickness skin grafts from the abdomen or groin for nipple-areolar complex creation. Areolas can be created by using a circular, full-thickness skin graft from the abdomen or groin, where the skin is slightly darker in color than the skin on the reconstructed breast. Three dimensional tattooing has become another popular modality of nipple areolar reconstruction, and the results are quite realistic and appealing to many patients (Figure 7).

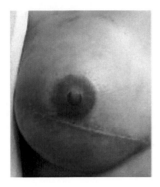

Figure 7. Nipple Areolar Three Dimensional Tattooing

OPTIONS FOR THE CONTRALATERAL BREAST

Some women elect to have bilateral mastectomy and reconstruction. By performing the same surgery on each breast, they are able to achieve pleasing symmetry. We have found that patients who chose bilateral mastectomy said they would make the same decision again compared to patients who chose unilateral mastectomy (Chen, presubmission).

If a unilateral mastectomy is performed on the involved breast, women have the option of various procedures on their healthy breast to achieve symmetry with their reconstruction. As mentioned earlier, this is a result of the Women's Health and Cancer Rights Act of 1998 (WHCRA), a federal law that requires insurers to cover surgery on the second breast if necessary for symmetry. The ultimate goal is for both the reconstructed breast and natural breast to have the same volume so that they can fit comfortably and symmetrically in a brassiere.

For women who are large breasted, a reduction of the healthy breast may be performed to match the reconstruction on the other side. Similarly, small-breasted women may elect for a breast augmentation on their natural breast to match their reconstruction (Figure 8). If the natural breast is ptotic, with sagging of the skin and breast tissue, a breast lift (mastopexy) can be performed to help match the reconstructed breast.

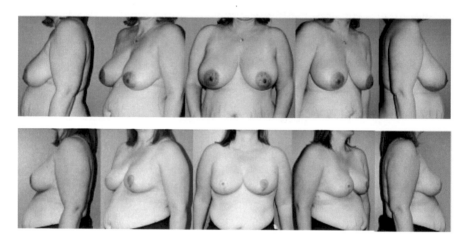

Figure 8. Unilateral Reconstruction with Balancing Procedure

Oncoplastic Reduction

This chapter focused on options for women undergoing total mastectomy. In women who undergo partial mastectomy, with or without radiation, combining the partial mastectomy with a breast reduction or mastopexy to prevent contour deformity, termed *oncoplastic reduction,* is an option. By rearranging the breast tissue after partial mastectomy, the plastic surgeon is able to create a pleasing new shape for both breasts. A candidate for oncoplastic reduction is someone with large, heavy breasts who suffers from chronic neck and back pain, shoulder grooving, and skin irritation in the inframammary folds (Figure 9). The oncoplastic reduction may be performed at the same time as the partial mastectomy, or in a second surgery shortly after, once final pathology has confirmed complete removal of the cancer with negative margins.

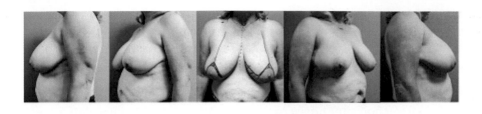

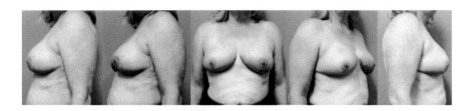

**Figure 9. Patient Marked for Oncoplastic Breast Reduction
and Postoperative Result**

Patients who have undergone prior partial mastectomy with radiation also may request reconstruction with a reduction or rearrangement technique months or years after their cancer treatment. Due to the radiation exposure, these patients are at increased risk of infection and wound healing complications, and an Omega pattern breast reduction technique is a safe alternative in these patients (Christiansen, 2008) (Figure 10).

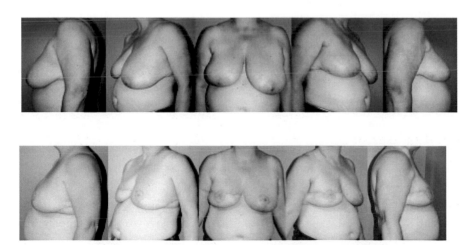

**Figure 10. Patient following Omega pattern breast reduction
performed after lumpectomy and radiation therapy**

CONCLUSION

Breast reconstruction is a very personal decision for each woman with breast cancer. The surgeon may guide the patient's decision-making process and provide information regarding specific options. Ultimately, the final decision to pursue breast reconstruction after breast cancer must be in line with each patient's values, lifestyle, and goals.

REFERENCES

1. Aeroform by AirXpanders. Patient-controlled tissue expansion. Accessed Dec 1, 2017. https://www.airxpanders.com/

2. Albornoz CR, Matros E, McCarthy CM, Klassen A, Cano SJ, Alderman AK, VanLaeken N, Lennox P, Macadam SA, Disa JJ, Mehrara BJ, Cordeiro PG, and Pusic AL (2014). Implant breast reconstruction and radiation: A multicenter analysis of long-term health-related quality of life and satisfaction. Ann Surg Oncol. 2014 Jul;21(7):2159-2164.

3. Centers for Medicare & Medicaid Services, Women's Health and Cancer Rights Act. Accessed Dec 1, 2017.https://www.cms.gov/CCIIO/Programs-and-Initiatives/Other-Insurance-Protections/whcra_factsheet.html.

4. Chen E, Langstein HN, and O'Connell A. Contralateral prophylactic mastectomy: the patient perspective. Pre-submission.

5. Christiansen D, Kazmier FR, and Puckett CL (2008). Safety and aesthetic improvement using the omega pattern reduction mammaplasty after breast conservation surgery and radiation therapy. Plastic and Reconstructive Surgery, 121(2):374-380.

6. Congress, H.R.2540 - Breast Cancer Patient Education Act of 2015. Accessed Dec 1, 2017. https://www.congress.gov/bill/114th-congress/house-bill/2540/text

7. Fischer JP, Nelson JA, Kovach SJ, Serletti JM, Wu LC, and Kanchwala S (2013). Impact of obesity on outcomes in breast reconstruction: Analysis of 15,937 patients from the ACS-NSQIP datasets. Journal of the American College of Surgeons, 217(4):656-664.

8. Jordan S, Khavanin N, and Kim J (2016). Seroma in prosthetic breast reconstruction. Plastic and Reconstructive Surgery, 137(4):1104–1116.

9. Krueger EA, Wilkins EG, Strawderman M, Cederna P, Goldfarb S, Vicini FA, and Pierce LJ (2001). Complications and patient satisfaction following expander/implant breast reconstruction with and without radiotherapy. International Journal of Radiation Oncology, Biology, and Physics, 49(3):713-721.

10. Loch-Wilkinson A, Beath KJ, Knight RJW, Wessels WLF, Magnusson M, Papadopoulos T, Connell T, Lofts J, Locke M, Hopper I, Cooter R, Vickery K, Joshi PA, Prince HM, and

Deva AK (2017). Breast Implant-Associated anaplastic large cell lymphoma in Australia and New Zealand: High-surface-area textured implants are associated with increased risk. <u>Plastic and Reconstructive Surgery</u>, 140(4):645-654.

11. Sbitany H, Piper M, and Lentz R (2017). Prepectoral breast reconstruction: A safe alternative to submuscular prosthetic reconstruction following nipple-sparing mastectomy. <u>Plastic and Reconstructive Surgery</u>, 140(3):432-443.

12. Sbitany H, Sandeen SN, Amalfi AN, Davenport MS, and Langstein HN (2009). Acellular dermis assisted prosthetic breast reconstruction versus complete submuscular coverage: A head to head comparison of outcomes. <u>Plastic and Reconstructive Surgery</u>, 124(6):1735-1740.

13. Sbitany H, Wang F, Peled AW, Lentz R, Alvarado M, Ewing CA, Esserman LJ, Fowble B, and Foster RD (2014). Immediate implant-based breast reconstruction following total skin-sparing mastectomy: Defining the risk of preoperative and postoperative radiation therapy for surgical outcomes. <u>Plastic and Reconstructive Surgery</u>, 134(3):396-404.

14. US Food and Drug Administration (2017a). Regulatory History of Breast Implants in the U.S. Accessed Dec 1, 2017. <u>https://www.fda.gov/MedicalDevices/ ProductsandMedicalProcedures/ImplantsandProsthetics/BreastImplants/ ucm064461.htm</u>

15. US Food and Drug Administration (2017b). Silicone Gel-Filled Breast Implants. Accessed Dec 1, 2017. <u>https://www.fda.gov/MedicalDevices/ProductsandMedicalProcedures/ ImplantsandProsthetics/BreastImplants/ucm063871.htm</u>

16. US Food and Drug Administration (2017c). Breast Implant-Associated Anaplastic Large Cell Lymphoma (BIA-ALCL). Accessed Dec 1, 2017. <u>https://www.fda.gov/ MedicalDevices/ProductsandMedicalProcedures/ImplantsandProsthetics/ BreastImplants/ucm239995.htm</u>

LIVING WITH BREAST CANCER

Hester Hill-Schnipper, L.I.C.S.W., BCD, OSW-C

INTRODUCTION

Life will never be quite the same as it was. This does not necessarily mean that it will be worse, just that it will be different. No matter the specifics of a breast cancer diagnosis, it rocks your world. For perhaps the first time, you are acutely aware of your mortality. Whatever the treatment, you have been challenged by physical hardships and probably some changes in your body. You consider all of your relationships and choices and may decide to make some changes. You value your time like never before, and you are acutely aware of how you spend it.

This chapter is about what it's like to live with breast cancer. The National Coalition of Cancer Survivors defines a survivor as anyone who has had a cancer diagnosis and counts it from that moment. Whether or not you agree with this definition, you now are part of this world. Your family and friends, no matter how much they love you, are unable to completely understand what you have been through. Part of your work is to educate them about the experience and your feelings.

In the next pages, we will talk about the usual course of the emotional/psychological side of having breast cancer. We also will discuss the most important issues facing us: relationships, spouses/partners and children, sexuality, professional concerns, financial worries, body image, anxiety, depression, and self-care.

CRISIS POINTS

There are known crisis points when you will feel particularly scared and sad and stressed. Understanding the predictability of these moments can help normalize them and help you more quickly return to a more comfortable mood.

Diagnosis: The first weeks after diagnosis are as tough as it ever gets psychologically. Whatever the details turn out to be, it is a little easier once there is a plan. In the very beginning, however, everyone feels panicked, very sad, and completely out of control. Am I going to die? How soon? What will happen to my children, to my family? Can I keep working? Who should I tell? Will I lose my breast(s)? Will I lose my hair? How will we pay for all of my care? Will I ever have a good night's sleep again?

Beginning Treatment: Treatment here refers to chemotherapy and/or radiation therapy. Radiation and chemotherapy often are more frightening than surgery, because they are unfamiliar and so closely tied to cancer. Once the treatment begins, however, people usually adapt fairly quickly and focus on getting through it.

Surgery, on the other hand, has a clear beginning and end. Many people also are understandably frightened by surgery, and women may have to make very tough choices about how much and what kind of surgery to treat the breast cancer. Once it's over, however, recovery usually happens slowly, surely, and steadily.

Losing your Hair: It is not vain or silly to be upset about being bald. Most treatments for early breast cancer cause alopecia/hair loss, and the process itself is distressing. Generally, it starts 14 to 20 days after the first round of chemotherapy. Some people have a 48-hour warning as their head starts to feel bruised all over; this is not like a headache, but rather a tenderness that is sore to the touch. If this happens, it means the hair is about to start falling, and the tenderness will resolve once it's gone.

Managing Hair Loss: The options regarding hair loss are: buzzing or shaving your head at about day 14, doing so immediately after the hair loss begins, or trying to hold onto each strand as long as possible. Decide what is best for you; have a wig and/or some scarves and hats at hand. Allow yourself to cry and scream and be generally angry and miserable. And then start to adapt. Hair almost always grows back after chemotherapy, and most women feel comfortable going out without a head covering about three months after the final treatment. Hair will then be short and chic.

Finishing Treatment: It seems counter-intuitive that this is a difficult transition, but many women find it harder than the treatment itself. They wonder: What happens now? If there are any cancer cells left, are they starting to grow? We also develop strong attachments to our caregivers and depend on seeing them regularly. It can be very frightening to suddenly go from daily radiation visits or weekly chemotherapy infusions to not seeing any healthcare provider for two or three months. Finally, it takes so much physical and emotional energy to get through cancer treatment that many women do not psychologically process the experience until it's done.

Recurrence: Fortunately, not everyone has to contend with this reality. If it happens, it often is even harder than the first diagnosis. Until now, it is possible to hope and believe that the cancer was gone. It can be overwhelming and terrifying to have to accept the reality that, while metastatic breast cancer can be treated, it cannot be cured. Since the focus of care for metastatic/advanced/stage IV breast cancer is containing it as long as possible, there is more attention paid to quality of life and how you are feeling day to day. The treatment itself may be physically easier than it was for early breast cancer (adjuvant therapy), but the emotional challenges often are greater.

Treatment Changes: The plan of treatment for advanced breast cancer is generally serial treatments. This means that you stay on any one therapy for as long as it is useful, and then a change is made. Unfortunately, cancer cells are very smart and eventually figure out how to resist any drug. Each time this happens, it may feel like a crisis as you wonder how many options remain. Be assured that there are many treatments available, and that the art and science of good cancer care means making the best choice at any given moment. After the new treatment has started and you are adjusted to any side effects and new rhythms, it gets easier.

Stopping Treatment: At some point, it becomes clear that the costs of anti-cancer therapies are greater than the benefits. The drugs may be making you sicker than the cancer itself, and stopping them can help you feel better. There have been studies that suggest that people who stop active treatment at this point may live longer than those who continue and have to contend with the risks and side effects of anti-cancer drugs.

End of Life: There is no way to make these feelings and days easy. Although we all know that we will die, and a cancer diagnosis brings that message loudly, the sadness and worry of this period are unique in their pain.

RELATIONSHIPS

We know that what really matters, what is most important in life, are our relationships. Cancer affects all of our most important connections in life. We worry about the people whom we love, and they worry about us.

Children

If we are parents, the most painful and intense concern is about our children. When we have children, we assume that we will live to raise them to adulthood. When that belief is called into question, we are terrified and devastated. First, remember that many women who are treated for breast cancer go on to live long and healthy lives and to dance at their children's weddings. There are a few guiding principles about talking with and caring for your children:

All children need honest, age-appropriate information. A six-year-old needs something different than a twelve-year-old, but they both need the truth.

When you talk with your children, and this is a continuing conversation, include these words: "This is not the time that you need to worry. If that time comes, I promise that I will tell you." And then do so.

Children need to have their routines kept as normal as possible. Reassure them that they can still go to soccer or ballet, and that someone will always be there to care for them.

Talk to your children's schools and tell them what is happening at home.

Include your children in your care as seems appropriate. It may be possible to take them with you to a short medical appointment and give them a tour of the place you receive care. At home, even a small child can bring you a glass of water or a sweater. Being straightforward about what is happening and about what helps will help normalize it.

Husbands/Partners

A breast cancer diagnosis is a major crisis for both partners. While your husband/ partner is, like you, sad and scared, he/she is also likely faced with managing more home responsibilities, continuing to work and bring in an income, and take care of you and your personal needs. Many partners find it very difficult to ask for help, and may need your assistance in organizing supports and resources. If, for example, there are long-standing issues between partners and their in-laws, they may flare up now. Everyone needs to find a way to step back, take a deep breath, and concentrate on the tasks at hand. Partners may also need encouragement to take time to be with friends or participate in activities that energize and fuel them.

Every couple has its own history and systems, but communication is vital. What do you need from each other? What are you most frightened about? How can you help one another best? What feels impossible?

Most couples depend on physical intimacy to help them get through hard times. Being close in this way reminds us of our love and mutual dependence. When intimacy seems daunting, this reliable strategy to get through pain may not be available. There will be more about this in a later section.

Other Family Members

Other family relationships may include parents, in-laws, siblings, and others. Each relationship is unique with expectations and wishes. No matter how old their child, parents are devastated if she is diagnosed with cancer. It can be hard to acknowledge their natural grief when all the attention is focused on the next generations. It helps if they can be genuinely helpful with childcare or household assistance. If that is not possible, try to identify other things they can do—even if that means frequent phone calls or sending checks to help with extra expenses.

Siblings also arrive at this moment with a history. If you have been close, this is a chance to be closer. If not, this is an opportunity for amends. Sadly, sometimes siblings do not deliver the hoped-for love and support.

Friends

There are always surprises about friendships. Some people whom you expect to be stellar supports will disappoint, and others will surprise you with their caring. Almost everyone loses at least one close friend through the cancer experience. It is obvious that this absence is due to their fear or other issues, but the reality is only of loss and hurt. Once cancer is behind you, you can decide whether it is worth the risk of an honest, painful conversation about your disappointment.

SEXUALITY AND INTIMACY

There are other chapters in this book that address the physical challenges of intimacy during and post breast cancer, so the focus here will be on the emotional components. We have all heard that the most important sexual organ is the brain, and it surely is changed during a cancer experience.

It is close to impossible to feel one's most beautiful, sexy, desirable, and womanly self while bald, nauseated, exhausted, and scared. No matter what your partner may tell you, the mirror and your body tell you something else. At the same time, you are in enormous need of tenderness and intimacy. If intercourse is not possible at any given time, there are other ways to love each other and feel close.

As always, it starts with honest communication. It feels terrible, when you love your partner, to withhold sex, but it can feel even worse to participate when you don't feel well. Put those feelings in words and listen to what he has to say, too. What do you both need right now? Sexual/physical release? Lying close, skin-to-skin? Feeling "held" and cherished and understood? Feeling safe? Sharing closeness in the way you do only with each other? If you can be very clear, you likely can find other ways to satisfy your desires.

You can enjoy back rubs or foot massages or holding hands while watching a movie. You can shower together. You can hold each other in bed while agreeing that sex is not part of the plan. You can whisper secrets and intimacies and honor the relationship that you share only with each other.

Especially if you have had a mastectomy, with or without reconstruction, your body has been changed. It is very important that your partner looks at and touches your chest or reconstructed breast as soon as it is physically comfortable. It usually is helpful to ask your partner to help with post-surgical care, such as emptying drains or helping you shower. Your new body will take some adjustment for you both, but the sooner it starts, the better. It is painful but important to talk about what you see and what you feel. For example, some women are devastated when, during sex, they see their partner's hand on a reconstructed breast, but can't feel it. Others are sad that their partner avoids the whole area. Talk about it.

If chemotherapy is part of your treatment, and, if that chemo results in sudden menopause, there will be a host of other issues that affect your intimate life. Again, these are addressed elsewhere in this book, but you must acknowledge and discuss them with your partner. You probably will need to relearn your body's responses, figure out what works for you now, and then teach your partner what you have learned.

PROFESSIONAL ISSUES

For many women, work often is a major part of self-identity, income, and social support. Making decisions about what to tell one's colleagues, whether or not to go to work through treatment, and how to return to work are all important questions. It is very helpful to have the flexibility and freedom to consider taking a medical or short-term leave. Many women, however, have jobs that don't include such benefits; if they don't work, they aren't paid.

Think carefully about these choices. If you work in a corporate environment, it may be helpful to speak with someone in human resources about your benefits and options before declaring your situation to your manager. If you don't work in such an environment, it may help to discuss the situation with a no-cost legal or government representative, such as one that may be found on the "Finding Legal Assistance" page of Cancer and Careers before you go public at work: http://www. cancerandcareers.org/en/at-work/legal-and-financial. Once you have shared the news, you can't take it back.

Cancer and Careers is a wonderful organization that can answer almost any questions you may have about work and cancer. Their main page is www. cancerandcareers.org

If you have the financial resources and work benefits to take a leave, think carefully about the choice. There likely are days when you can't work, e.g., right after surgery or the first few days after a chemotherapy infusion, but there are others when you will feel well enough to do so. You may be able to simply use your sick leave or vacation time. Some jobs, however, are so demanding physically or pressured or stressful that they are impossible to do during cancer treatment. Others can be a source of distraction and normalcy. Perhaps working less than full time for a period of time is an option you could discuss with your employer.

FINANCES

Cancer is expensive. There are deductibles and co-pays and uncovered medical bills. There likely are higher costs for gas and parking and extended childcare hours or other household help. There may well be reduced income. There are no perfect solutions to these problems, but there are many organizations that can be helpful. You can start by asking to speak with a social worker at the hospital or cancer center where you are treated. You also can look at resources online; good places to start are Cancer Care (https://www.cancercare.org/) or Living Beyond Breast Cancer (http://www.lbbc.org/). Both excellent organizations have useful resources and guides related to financial issues.

ANXIETY AND DEPRESSION

Anxiety and depression are normal responses to breast cancer and its aftermath. Everyone is scared, and everyone is sad. It is important to discern how to understand normal reactions to a difficult situation vs. depression or anxiety that needs extra professional help and, perhaps, medication.

The prevalence of mental illness among cancer patients mirrors that of the general population. Since cancer patients come from all walks of life, there will be some who begin with pre-existing mental illness, depression, anxiety, and/or substance abuse. Others, who have been managing satisfactorily, will become less emotionally stable and be unable to adequately cope with the diagnosis of a life-threatening illness.

Although many people with cancer struggle with depression and/or anxiety, especially shortly after diagnosis and at other times of heightened crisis, it is important to note that most manage the many stresses of a cancer diagnosis and treatment without requiring special assistance. Although feelings of sadness, grief, and anxiety are very common, they usually subside in time with the support of extended family, friends, and caregivers.

It is estimated that approximately 25% of cancer patients and survivors struggle with depression. The incidence of anxiety is similar. There are differences between a clinical depression that will likely respond to medication and a normal reaction to a difficult and stressful situation. Except for people who have extraordinary denial, an adjustment reaction with mixed feelings is almost a given. Remember that sadness and worry are not signs of a psychiatric disorder: emotional lability or a shorter than usual temper do not automatically mean that someone needs psychopharmacologic assistance. It is difficult to tease out symptoms of major depression from those normally associated with cancer treatment and recovery. The usual symptom list, including difficulties with sleep and appetite, fatigue, reduced interest in usual activities and relationships, difficulty with concentration, and a sense of being out of control, is just as relevant for normal reactions to cancer treatment as it is for depression.

How do you know if your feelings are more than a normal reaction to a difficult time and that seeing a therapist would be helpful?

If your feelings of sadness or anxiety are interfering with your ability to manage your days, if you are not sleeping or awakening too often at night or awakening at 3 AM and being up for the duration, if you are crying or feeling numb most days, if you feel hopeless and can't identify things that you are looking forward to, and if these feelings have persisted for more than a month or six weeks, it is time to talk with a professional.

Choosing the right therapist means more than finding someone who takes your insurance and has openings at a time and place that is convenient. It also means finding someone who is experienced with people who have/have had cancer. You don't want to spend valuable therapy dollars and time educating someone about the experience. Finally, it is of critical importance to like and respect your therapist. As in all human relationships, the connection and chemistry matter.

POST TRAUMATIC STRESS SYNDROME

Post-Traumatic Stress Syndrome (PTSS) can be a useful way to frame your feelings and reactions. Initially used to describe a syndrome seen in soldiers returning from war, the diagnosis has been expanded to include people coping after any traumatic event. The symptoms include ruminating about the experience, remembering and reliving the details and moments, avoiding places that remind you of the experience, difficulty with sleep, feeling badly about yourself, feeling vulnerable or on high alert, physical (somatic) symptoms that don't have an obvious cause, problems with relationships, and difficulty controlling your feelings.

These feelings are a frequent accompaniment to cancer and cancer survivorship, but they can be so intense that they interfere with your personal and work lives. If so, this is a time to find the right therapist.

SELF IMAGE

Body issues and self-esteem are concerns for most women during and after breast cancer. There may have been permanent changes from cancer surgeries, and there may be other temporary changes like alopecia and weight gain. The reality is that it takes time to adjust to and accept one's new physical self. Given the emphasis on youth and good looks in our culture, it is painful to feel that both have been lost through the course of illness and treatment. The first flush of euphoria about completing treatment and being alive fades quickly, and one is left with a body that may look and feel unfamiliar. Gained weight usually can be lost through a disciplined program of diet and exercise. It also is important to remember that the pounds may hang on tenaciously, and that the more important goals are fitness and improved energy.

SELF CARE

The obvious suggestions about getting enough sleep, eating well, seeing friends, and treating yourself to small luxuries hold. However, there is much more to healthy self-care after cancer. It can be a struggle to learn to again trust your body. The shock of facing mortality and learning to live without promises of health may be daunting.

It is clear that the best goal is to live as though the cancer will never return. If it does, it will not have been helpful to spend the intervening months or years feeling sad and scared. If it does, you will have to deal with it then, and there really is no advantage to trying to prepare.

This is the moment to start putting yourself and your own needs first—at least some of the time. You no longer have to settle for the smallest slice of chocolate cake, literally or figuratively. Consciously try to express your wishes and make them happen.

Cancer forces you to step away from the busy demands of life, at least for a time, and this presents an opportunity to contemplate choices. Some women leave unhappy marriages or relationships and others move to a permanent commitment.

Some women make career changes, and virtually everyone makes small changes in friendships and routines. Accepting that life is finite can be a positive force for happiness.

It can be helpful to imagine an emotional bank account. Life requires some withdrawals, but you now have an absolute need to make deposits. What makes you happy? Who makes you laugh? Where and how do you like to spend your free time?

The best self-care means being as kind to yourself as you are to those whom you love.

CANCER SURVIVORSHIP

Michael T. Milano, M.D., Ph.D. and Michelle Shayne, M.D.

INTRODUCTION

Cancer survivorship has developed into an integral component of cancer management. Survivorship care entails informing the patient of the treatment she has received, possible consequences of treatment, and a follow-up plan. Educating the patient on her treatment involves providing her with a treatment care summary—a one to two page outline of the treatment received and planned (i.e., several years of hormonal therapy), that can be shared with primary care and other providers. A care plan also should be provided, detailing the strategy for: (1) cancer surveillance, (2) identifying and managing treatment-related late effects, (3) promoting healthy lifestyles and preventative care, and (4) facilitating referral to ancillary care services to assist with late complications and psychosocial/quality of life concerns.

While cancer can be a deadly disease, the number of cancer survivors continues to increase, in part due to earlier cancer screening and detection, improved cancer treatment options, and an aging population. The number of breast cancer survivors in the United States (U.S.) population in 2016 was estimated to be 3.6 million (among more than 15 million total cancer survivors) with projections of 4.6 million (of 20 million total cancer survivors) by 2026 (Miller, 2016). Many of these breast cancer survivors will have received radiation therapy, depending on their age, stage, extent of resection, and type (i.e., histologic and pathologic characteristics); many will have been cured of breast cancer. In one study, there were a total of 1.25 million radiation-treated breast cancer survivors in the U.S. (representing 40% of the total number of radiation-treated cancer survivors) with projected increases to two million in 2030 (Bryant, 2017). In another study, the total number of breast cancer patients (including invasive and in-situ disease) receiving a first course of radiation therapy is expected to increase from 133,000 to 156,000 (among 490,000 to 580,000 total patients) annually from 2015 to 2025, accounting for projected cancer incidence and population increases (Pan, 2016).

The treatments for breast cancer can have immediate adverse effects (referred to as acute toxicities), as well as late adverse effects (late toxicities or late effects), which can occur months to years after diagnosis and treatment of the cancer. Cancer treatments, including surgery, radiation therapy, chemotherapy, and hormonal therapy all can cause late effects. Surgery and radiation are considered local treatment modalities, meaning that these interventions target a specific part of the body and, as a result, the late adverse effects from these treatment modalities tend to be within the region treated. The adverse effects from systemic agents (i.e., chemotherapy, biologic drug therapy, hormonal therapy) can occur in tissue remote from the tumor. For example, the chemotherapeutic agent, doxorubicin, can cause cardiac toxicity even years after treatment has been completed. Some of the newer agents that potentiate an immunologic response against cancer can cause inflammatory (i.e., pulmonary pneumonitis) or autoimmune reactions.

Late adverse effects are a result of several possible factors, including tissue removal (i.e., surgical resection of lymph nodes), tissue disruption, tissue destruction, disruption of tissue vascularity (i.e., small vessels that provide blood flow), and/or fibrosis (scarring). Altered tissue or organ function would need to be clinically detectable to be considered a late adverse effect; these effects would be apparent from symptomology and/or quantitative clinical assessment (examples being pulmonary function tests, echocardiogram, neurocognitive assessment tools). It often is not possible to distinguish adverse treatment-related effects from effects directly related to the initial cancer (i.e., from tumor infiltration into normal tissues) or from causes unrelated to the cancer or cancer treatment (i.e., poor cardiopulmonary function from chronic smoking).

There are several scoring and grading systems to quantify the extent of these toxicities. One such scoring system is the National Cancer Institute/National Institutes of Health Common Terminology Criteria for Adverse Events (CTCAE); the latest version is available online: https://ctep.cancer.gov/protocoldevelopment/electronic_applications/ctc.htm

Toxicities are graded based upon the specific sign or symptom and the severity of the sign or symptom. Generally, grade 1 toxicities are mild and do not require intervention; grade 2 toxicities require minor interventions; grade 3 toxicities are of moderate severity, requiring moderate-to major-interventions; grade 4 toxicities are life-threatening; and grade 5 toxicities represent fatality from the toxicity. The CTCAE does not classify toxicities based upon the timing of the toxicity (i.e., it does not differentiate acute versus late toxicities) nor does it ascribe a cause for the toxicity (i.e., it does not assign toxicities as due to radiation, surgery, or chemotherapy).

Chemotherapy and/or radiation therapy may result in second malignancies, because radiation and many chemotherapeutic agents are carcinogenic (Travis, 2011). For radiation therapy, the risks of cancer induction are related to the radiation dose delivered, the body region(s) exposed to radiation, the age of the patient, and possibly genetic susceptibilities of the patient to cancer induction (Hindorff, 2011, and Brooks, 2012). Radiation-induced cancers, when they do occur, generally develop within the previous radiation field more than five years, but often decades after radiation.

Adult survivors of childhood cancer have unique issues related to a greater susceptibility to treatment-related effects, longer lifespan after the diagnosis and treatment of cancer, and adverse late effects related to compromised growth and development, specifically bone growth, sexual maturation, and neurocognitive development. Children are more susceptible to treatment-induced second malignancies, including breast cancer, which can appear in adulthood. Hodgkin's lymphoma survivors treated with radiation at a young age are at a particularly greater risk of breast cancer and are more apt to die from breast cancer (or other cancers) after breast cancer diagnosis than women in the general population (Milano, 2010).

Most of the remainder of this chapter will focus on treatment-induced late effects relevant to patients who developed cancer as adults. The acute effects of treatment are discussed briefly as well, as severe acute toxicity also can have long-standing effects.

It is noteworthy that some women (and men) with so-called "incurable" breast cancer can live many years. Not falling within the classic category of "survivor," many prefer to be called a cancer thriver—someone living with an incurable, but manageable, disease. The issues of acute and late effects from treatment that are discussed here are relevant to them as well.

ACUTE TREATMENT-RELATED EFFECTS

Surgery, radiation, and drug therapy can have acute effects occurring during, or shortly after therapy.

Post-surgical risks depend on the type and extent of resection. Women can undergo breast-conserving resection in which a portion of the breast is removed, or mastectomy, of which there are various types, depending on the extent of other tissue removed in addition to the breast and overlying skin/nipple (i.e., in addition to what is removed with a simple mastectomy). For example, a modified radical mastectomy implies the additional removal of axillary (underarm) lymph nodes. Some women may undergo a sentinel node dissection in which one or few nodes, identified as being highest risk, are removed. Women who undergo a mastectomy may undergo reconstruction (discussed in the chapter "Breast Reconstruction: Knowing the Options"). Post-reconstruction risks depend on the timing and type of reconstruction performed. As with any surgery, acute risks include bleeding, infection, and poor wound healing.

Toxicities are common among women undergoing radiation that is either acute (occurring during radiation treatment) or subacute (occurring in the weeks to months after radiation treatment). These commonly include fatigue and skin desquamation, characterized by a spectrum ranging from mild erythema and/or dry flaking skin within the radiation field to moist peeling skin, either in patches (commonly under the breast) or more confluent. Ulceration, hemorrhage, and necrosis are much rarer complications. The skin may be treated to high doses intentionally in order to best treat the cancer, with the most common scenario being the delivery of radiation to the chest wall and scar after mastectomy.

For systemic therapy, including chemotherapy, acute toxicity is variable depending on the drugs used. Common chemotherapy-related toxicity includes fatigue/malaise, hair loss, nausea, vomiting, hematologic toxicity (including anemia, susceptibilities to infection, and/or bleeding), diarrhea, constipation, mucositis, peripheral neuropathy (including numbness, tingling, and/or pain), and skin and nail changes. Disruption in kidney and/or liver function can be observed as well. Most, though not all, of these acute toxicities from chemotherapy are reversible.

Acute effects of endocrine (hormonal) therapy for breast cancer most commonly include hot flashes, headache, stomach upset, skin rash, joint and muscle pain, depression, and cough. These effects usually resolve after the drug is held for two to three weeks. Interestingly, acute side effects experienced when on one of the three currently available aromatase inhibitors may not be experienced by the same individual when on another agent within the same class. This allows patients to try another equally effective endocrine therapy that may be better tolerated, despite its identical mechanism of action. The reason for this is not completely understood (Brit, 2010).

LATE TREATMENT-RELATED EFFECTS ORGANIZED BY ORGAN SYSTEM

Skin and Soft Tissue

Generally, post-treatment late skin and soft tissue effects are mild in nature. Severe, late skin and soft tissue post-treatment (surgical and radiation) effects generally are uncommon and include ulceration, wound dehiscence, disfiguring scarring, and fibrosis. All patients undergoing external beam radiation are treated with radiation beams that go through skin and soft tissue. Historically (before 1960), the skin was the dose-limiting organ in the treatment of cancer with radiation. Many patients would develop severe desquamation and ulceration of the skin, necessitating premature completion of radiation treatment. Those patients who survived would develop telangiectasia, dense dermal fibrosis, sebaceous gland atrophy, loss of hair follicles, altered melanin deposition, and skin ulceration. In the modern era, the radiation beams are more penetrating (due to higher energy) and able to be delivered in a more conformal manner (i.e., shaped to the breast or chest wall contour; discussed in more detail later); therefore, skin reactions generally are less toxic than they had been in previous decades.

Breast cancer survivors also are at risk for developing lymphedema—a mild to potentially debilitating swelling of the hand and arm on the same side as the treated breast cancer. Lymphedema typically is the result of axillary node dissection, with risks increased in women who have bulky nodal disease, extensive nodal dissection, and/or axillary radiation. This topic is covered in more detail in the chapter The Biology and Management of Lymphedema in the Breast Cancer Patient."

Lung

The breast is situated over the chest wall (comprising ribs; sternum; pectoralis muscles, and intercostal muscles, and nerves between the ribs) in a convex manner. Directly under the chest wall are the lungs. Thus, when treating the chest wall or breast, the underlying lung is exposed to radiation as well. The lung tissue has a relatively low threshold for radiation-induced damage, with respect to development of pneumonitis (an inflammatory condition resulting in dyspnea, cough, and low-grade fever) and subsequent fibrosis/scarring. Radiation can impair pulmonary function—specifically the diffusion capacity and forced expiratory volumes measured by testing. These complications are correlated directly with the volume of lung exposed to supra-threshold doses of radiation (Marks, 2010). Patients with normal lung function prior to treatment may not be symptomatic from post-radiation fibrosis. More modern radiation techniques (discussed in the cardiac section) more effectively spare the lung from radiation.

Chemotherapy agents (not typically used for breast cancer), such as bleomycin and the nitrosoureas, can produce severe lung toxicities. Bleomycin is associated with pulmonary fibrosis and decreased diffusion capacity. Management of cancer treatment-related lung disease is the same as the management of pulmonary-related disease in the general population. Patients at risk of cancer treatment-related toxicity should be counseled for prevention of pulmonary decline (i.e., smoking cessation and exercise).

Heart

After radiation exposure to the heart, cardiac toxicity can develop, often years to decades after the exposure (Travis, 2011). The spectrum of clinical manifestations of cardiac injury mirrors specific cardiac syndromes for which the general population is at risk, including coronary artery disease, pericarditis, cardiomyopathy, valvular damage, and/or arrhythmias. These late effects are correlated directly to the heart dose and volume of heart (primarily the left ventricle) exposed to radiation (Gagliardi, 2010, and Sardar, 2017). From a Swedish/Danish study of 960 breast cancer survivors (treated from 1958 to 2001) who experienced major coronary events, along with 1,205 controls, there was a linear relationship with mean radiation dose to the heart and coronary events (Darby, 2013). Unexpectedly, no threshold dose (i.e., dose below which there is no risk) was apparent. Notably, these findings may not necessarily apply to women treated with modern radiation planning and delivery methods. A similar trend, albeit lower risk, was reported in a recent analysis of 40,781 women (among 75 published studies) treated with either no radiation or radiation delivered with more modern radiation doses and techniques (Taylor, 2017). Continued efforts are being made to develop novel approaches and technologies to reduce heart and lung dose exposure in women undergoing radiation for breast cancer. These include: (1) modulating the beam such that the dose is shaped more conformally (termed intensity-modulated radiation), (2) proton beam radiation therapy (a form of radiation that is less penetrating into normal tissues), (3) prone radiation (woman laying on her belly, with the breasts hanging through a board, allowing for greater separation of the treated breast from the chest wall), (4) partial breast radiation (as opposed to whole breast radiation) for women with low-risk disease, (5) the use of breath hold techniques that allow for some separation of the breast and chest wall from the heart, while minimizing motion during treatment, and (6) gating of the radiation, meaning that the treatment is delivered only when the breast is in a certain position during the normal respiratory cycle (or during shallow breathing).

Certain chemotherapy agents also result in cardiac toxicity; anthracyclines are the best-recognized cardiotoxic chemotherapy agents z9 (Gagliardi, 2010). Human epidermal growth factor receptor2 (Her2) targeted therapies such as trastuzumab (Herceptin®) and pertuzumab are biologic drugs (antibodies) also associated with cardiac toxicity. Management of radiation- and chemotherapy-related cardiac disease is the same as the management of cardiac-related disease in the general population, although patients at risk of cancer treatment-related toxicity should be screened regularly with stress testing and should be counseled for prevention (i.e., smoking cessation, diet, and exercise).

Some endocrine therapy, which is ideally continued for at least a five-year duration, is associated rarely with angina pectoris and myocardial infarction. Presumably, this is due, at least in part, to the effects aromatase inhibitors can exert on cholesterol metabolism. It is important that patients on aromatase inhibition undergo routine surveillance of cholesterol levels and undergo appropriate interventions to address dyslipidemia, whether dietary, exercise-, or medication-mediated.

Reproductive Endocrine

Alkylating chemotherapy agents, as well as gonadal radiation (generally not relevant to breast cancer survivors) can impair ovarian function. Late effects from adult female ovarian damage include infertility, oligomenorrhea/amenorrhea, hot flashes, atrophic vulvitis and vaginitis, changes in fat distribution, breast changes, bone demineralization, and diminished libido. Infertility can be multifactorial (Nieman, 2006). The chapter "Fertility Preservation and Cancer Care" covers this topic in greater detail.

Bone

High doses of radiation (for example of the ribs underlying the breast) can result in increased risk of bone fracture, chest wall pain, and (rarely) bone necrosis. Patients receiving bisphosphonates for bone metastases or bone metastases prevention (Coleman, 2015) are at risk of bone osteonecrosis (most commonly in the jaw but also other sites such as the femur). Newer agents such as denosumab (which inhibit osteoclast maturation) pose similar risks (Melisko, 2016). Aromatase inhibitors (a type of hormonal agent) are associated with greater risks of osteopenia, osteoporosis, and fractures.

Bone Marrow

Most chemotherapeutic drugs (with the exception of some, though not all, biologic agents) suppress bone marrow with the extent of suppression based upon the specific chemotherapy agent and dosing scheme. Radiation also is bone marrow suppressing but only to the extent to which bone marrow is in the radiation field (and very little bone marrow is present in the ribs or clavicle). Bone marrow suppression primarily is an acute toxicity, although late marrow suppression is possible, generally to a much lesser extent than what occurs acutely. The lumbosacral spine and pelvis account for most of the active marrow— for example, in patients undergoing concurrent chemotherapy and radiation therapy for gynecologic malignancies, newer technologies of radiation are used to relatively spare the pelvic bone marrow (Mell, 2017).

Alkylating agents and anthracycline chemotherapeutic agents have been associated with an increased risk of leukemia as a late effect of treatment. Alkylating, agent-related

128

acute leukemia characteristically develops following an average latency period of five to seven years, and overt leukemia is many times preceded by a myelodysplastic phase (Azim, 2011). In contrast, anthracycline agent-related leukemia arises after a typically much shorter latency period of about two years, and the secondary leukemias which arise after anthracyclines tend to have no previous myelodysplastic phase (Smith, 2003). An analysis of several adjuvant studies conducted by the National Surgical Adjuvant Breast and Bowel Project group using chemotherapy regimens containing both doxorubicin, an anthracycline, and cyclophosphamide, an alkylating agent, reported a five-year incidence of leukemia ranging from 0.3% to 1.2% (Smith, 2003).

Granulocyte colony stimulating factors (G-CSF) often are used to decrease the myelosuppressive effects of chemotherapy. The potential association between G-CSF and secondary leukemia after treatment for breast cancer is debated, although in-vitro data suggest G-CSF may increase the risk of leukemia and myelodysplasia. One SEER-Medicare, population-based analysis of women with breast cancer treated with adjuvant chemotherapy, found G-CSF use was associated with a doubling in the risk of secondary leukemia or myelodysplasia compared with chemotherapy delivered without the growth factor. The risk of these secondary malignancies in that study for patients who received growth factors within 48 months of diagnosis was 1.8% compared to 0.7% of patients who did not receive growth factors (hazard ratio = 2.59, 95% CI = 1.30 to 5.15) (Hershman, 2007).

Nervous System

Women undergoing chemotherapy for breast cancer can experience what commonly is referred to as "chemobrain" in which cognition is impaired (Hermelink, 2015). These women may benefit from neurocognitive assessment and rehabilitation. This topic is discussed in greater detail in the chapter "Relationships between Cognitive Impairments in Breast Cancer Survivors and Menopause."

Some chemotherapy agents (including taxanes) can cause peripheral neuropathy, in which patients experience pain and/or numbness in the extremities (Schneider, 2015; Gewandter, 2017; Staff, 2017). Currently, pharmacologic management remains the standard of care; a 2014 practice guideline concluded that the best evidence supported a benefit from the drug duloxetine, although others (such as tricyclic antidepressants, gabapentin, a compounded topical gel of baclofen, amitriptyline, and ketamine) could be considered given the limited treatment options (Hershman, 2014).

The cochlea and, therefore, hearing, also is susceptible to treatment-related damage; this is a common effect of platinum-based chemotherapy; radiation to the cochlea also can impair hearing (Bhandare, 2010). Tamoxifen (a hormonal agent) increases the risk of forming blood clots, which can result in deep venous thrombosis, pulmonary embolism, and stroke. The frequency of both venous and arterial thromboses was 5.4% among patients who received tamoxifen therapy and 1.6% among patients on observation (p=.0002) in one analysis of seven consecutive Eastern Cooperative Oncology Group (ECOG) studies of adjuvant therapy for breast cancer and associated risk of vascular complications (Saphner, 1991).

Kidney

A variety of chemotherapy agents have been implicated as renal toxic, particularly platinum-based drugs. The management of cancer treatment-induced kidney disease is the same as the management of kidney disease in the general population, including low protein diet, fluid and salt restrictions, dialysis, and renal transplantation.

SECOND MALIGNANCIES

There are abundant data that cancer survivors are at an increased risk of second malignancies (Dores, 2002, and Travis, 2011). Chemotherapy and/or radiation therapy potentially are carcinogenic as a result of DNA damage and, therefore, are implicated as a major cause of second cancer induction. Tamoxifen (a hormonal agent) increases the risk of endometrial (uterine) cancer; women receiving this drug are recommended to undergo regular Pap smears and ultrasound or selective endometrial biopsies.

Cancer patients may have inherent genetic susceptibility to develop additional cancers. Treatment-induced cancers generally occur many years to decades following treatment. Radiation-induced cancers occur within the previously treated radiation field, while chemotherapy-induced cancers can occur anywhere in the body. Patients are susceptible not only to solid tumor cancers (such as breast, lung, colon) but also leukemia and lymphoma. An increased risk of lung cancer after treatment for breast cancer is well-described in the literature (Milano, 2014, and Taylor, 2017). Breast cancer survivors also are at greater risk of developing a second breast cancer, with risks increased by contralateral breast radiation exposure (much reduced using modern techniques) (Taylor, 2017) and reduced from prolonged (several year) hormonal therapy. Generally, it is recommended that cancer survivors maintain a healthy, cancer-preventative lifestyle (i.e., no tobacco use, healthy diet, exercise) and undergo regular clinical examination and screening examinations (i.e., mammography and colonoscopy).

PSYCHOSOCIAL/QUALITY OF LIFE

There is growing awareness of the psychosocial issues facing cancer survivors, including psychologic/psychiatric symptoms (including anxiety, depression, guilt, shame) (Mitchell, 2013; Andersen, 2014; Lang, 2015; and McDonnell, 2015); body-related shame after potentially disfiguring therapy (Castonguay, 2017); financial difficulty related to costs of treatment and follow-up, as well as potential loss of employment/underemployment (Kiasuwa, 2016; Rim, 2016; Bilodeau, 2017; and Catt, 2017) generalized lack of social well-being (Catt, 2017); and sexual dysfunction (Krychman, 2006; Dizon, 2014; and Zhou, 2015). Patient and provider awareness of these issues, as well as availability of resources to address these issues, are critical to survivorship care. Also important is the promotion of healthy lifestyles, including smoking cessation (Duan, 2017), regular exercise (Doyle, 2006; Rock, 2012; Mustian, 2013; Mustian, 2016; Swartz, 2017; and Zhang, 2017), and a healthy, balanced diet (Doyle, 2006; Rock, 2012; Ladas, 2014; and Zhang, 2017). Integrative (i.e., complementary, alternative) therapies such as massage may play a role in addressing physical and emotional effects of cancer and cancer therapy, although they remain under-studied. Growing evidence suggests potential benefits from mind-body therapies including acupressure, acupuncture, music therapy, meditation, relaxation, stress management, and yoga; while dietary supplements also may provide some benefit, little data support their use (Greenlee, 2017).

CONCLUSION

The recently published "American Cancer Society/American Society of Clinical Oncology Breast Cancer Survivorship Care Guideline" exhaustively reviewed evidence-based guidelines for breast cancer survivorship (Runowicz, 2016a, and Runowicz, 2016b) and is a useful tool for healthcare professionals. These guidelines ranked (based upon level of evidence) the recommendations on frequency and type of assessments for breast cancer recurrence and late treatment-related complications (many of which are discussed above).

Fortunately, there has been a great effort devoted to understanding the issues facing women (and men) who are breast cancer survivors and developing strategies to keep the patient and primary care providers informed of what treatment was given and what impact that might have on the patient in both the near and distant future. Further work is needed to refine evidence-based recommendations for patients, such that optimal, cost-effective care is given to cancer survivors. Much work has been done, and more work needs to follow!

REFERENCES

1. Andersen BL, DeRubeis RJ, Berman BS, Gruman J, Champion VL, Massie MJ, Holland JC, Partridge AH, Bak K, Somerfield MR, and Rowland JH (2014). Screening, assessment, and care of anxiety and depressive symptoms in adults with cancer: An American Society of Clinical Oncology guideline adaptation. Journal of Clinical Oncology, 32(15):1605-1619.

2. Azim HA, Jr., de Azambuja E, Colozza M, Bines J, and Piccart MJ (2011). Long-term toxic effects of adjuvant chemotherapy in breast cancer. Annals of Oncology, 22(9):1939-1947.

3. Bhandare N, Jackson A, Eisbruch A, Pan CC, Flickinger JC, Antonelli P, and Mendenhall WM (2010). Radiation Therapy and Hearing Loss. International Journal of Radiation Oncology, Biology, and Physics, 76:S50-S57.

4. Bilodeau K, Tremblay D, and Durand MJ (2017). Exploration of return-to-work interventions for breast cancer patients: A scoping review. Supportive Care in Cancer, 25.10.1007/s00520-016-3526-2.

5. Briot K, Tubiana-Hulin M, Bastit L, Kloos I, and Roux C (2010). Effect of a switch of aromatase inhibitors on musculoskeletal symptoms in postmenopausal women with hormone-receptor-positive breast cancer: the ATOLL (articular tolerance of letrozole) study. Breast Cancer Research and Treatment,120(1):127-134.

6. Brooks JD, Teraoka SN, Reiner AS, Satagopan JM, Bernstein L, Thomas DC, Capanu M, Stovall M, Smith SA, Wei S, Shore RE, Boice JD Jr, Lynch CF, Mellemkjaer L, Malone KE, Liang X; Wecare Study Collaborative Group, Haile RW, Concannon P, and Bernstein JL (2012). Variants in activators and downstream targets of ATM, radiation exposure, and contralateral breast cancer risk in the WECARE study. Human Mutation, 33(1):158-164.

7. Bryant AK, Banegas MP, Martinez ME, Mell LK, and Murphy JD (2017). Trends in radiation therapy among cancer survivors in the United States, 2000-2030. Cancer Epidemiology, Biomarkers, and Prevention, 26(6):963-970.

8. Castonguay AL, Wrosch C, Pila E, and Sabiston CM (2017). Body-related shame and guilt predict physical activity in breast cancer survivors over time. Oncology Nursing Forum, 44(4):465-475.

9. Catt S, Starkings R, Shilling V, and Fallowfield L (2017). Patient-reported outcome measures of the impact of cancer on patients' everyday lives: A systematic review. Journal of Cancer Survivorship, 11(2):211-232.

10. Darby SC, Ewertz M, McGale P, Bennet AM, Blom-Goldman U, Brønnum D, Correa C, Cutter D, Gagliardi G, Gigante B, Jensen MB, Nisbet A, Peto R, Rahimi K, Taylor C, and Hall P (2013). Risk of ischemic heart disease in women after radiotherapy for breast cancer. New England Journal of Medicine, 368:987-998.

11. Dizon DS, Suzin D, and McIlvenna S (2014). Sexual health as a survivorship issue for female cancer survivors. Oncologist, 19:202-210.

12. Dores GM, Metayer C, Curtis RE, Lynch CF, Clarke EA, Glimelius B, Storm H, Pukkala E, van Leeuwen FE, Holowaty EJ, Andersson M, Wiklund T, Joensuu T, van't Veer MB, Stovall M, and Gospodarowicz M (2002). Second malignant neoplasms among long-term survivors of Hodgkin's disease: A population-based evaluation over 25 years. Journal of Clinical Oncology, 20(16):3484-3494.

13. Doyle C, Kushi LH, Byers T, Courneya KS, Demark-Wahnefried W, Grant B, McTiernan A, Rock CL, Thompson C, Gansler T, and Andrews KS (2006). Nutrition and physical activity during and after cancer treatment: An American Cancer Society guide for informed choices. CA: A Cancer Journal for Clinicians, 56(6):323-353.

14. Duan W, Li S, Meng X, Sun Y, and Jia C (2017). Smoking and survival of breast cancer patients: A meta-analysis of cohort studies. Breast, 33:117-124.

15. Early Breast Cancer Trialists' Collaborative Group, Coleman R, Powles T, et al. (2015). Adjuvant bisphosphonate treatment in early breast cancer: Meta-analyses of individual patient data from randomised trials. Lancet, 386:1353-1361.

16. Gagliardi G, Constine LS, Moiseenko W, Correa C, Pierce LJ, Allen AM, and Marks LB (2010). Radiation-associated heart injury. International Journal of Radiation Oncology Biology and Physics, 76(3):S77-S85.

17. Gewandter JS, Freeman R, Kitt RA, Cavaletti G, Gauthier LR, McDermott MP, Mohile NA, Mohlie SG, Smith AG, Tejani MA, Turk DC, and Dworkin RH (2017). Chemotherapy-induced peripheral neuropathy clinical trials: Review and recommendations. Neurology, 89(8):859-869.

18. Greenlee H, DuPont-Reyes MJ, Balneaves LG, Carlson LE, Cohen MR, Deng G, Johnson JA, Mumber M, Seely D, Zick SM, Boyce LM, and Tripathy D (2017). Clinical practice guidelines on the evidence-based use of integrative therapies during and after breast cancer treatment. CA: Cancer Journal for Clinicians, 67(3):194-232.

19. Hermelink K (2015). Chemotherapy and cognitive function in breast cancer patients: The so-called chemo brain. Journal of the National Cancer Institute. Monographs, (51):67-69.

20. Hershman D, Neugut AI, Jacobson JS, Wang J, Tsai WY, McBride R, Bennett CL, and Grann VR (2007). Acute myeloid leukemia or myelodysplastic syndrome following use of granulocyte colony-stimulating factors during breast cancer adjuvant chemotherapy. Journal of the National Cancer Institute, 99(3):196-205.

21. Hershman DL, Lacchetti C, Dworkin RH, Lavoie Smith EM, Bleeker J, Cavaletti G, Chauhan C, Gavin P, Lavino A, Lustberg MB, Paice J, Schneider B, Smith ML, Smith T, Terstriep S, Wagner-Johnston N, Bak K, and Loprinzi CL (2014). Prevention and management of chemotherapy-induced peripheral neuropathy in survivors of adult cancers: American Society of Clinical Oncology clinical practice guideline. Journal of Clinical Oncology, 32(18):1941-1967.

22. Hindorff LA, Gillanders EM, and Manolio TA (2011). Genetic architecture of cancer and other complex diseases: Lessons learned and future directions. Carcinogenesis, 32(7):945-954.

23. Kiasuwa Mbengi R, Otter R, Mortelmans K, Arbyn M, Van Oyen H, Bouland C, and de Brouwer C (2016). Barriers and opportunities for return-to-work of cancer survivors: Time for action--rapid review and expert consultation. Systematic Reviews, 5:35.

24. Krychman ML, Pereira L, Carter J, and Amsterdam A (2006). Sexual oncology: Sexual health issues in women with cancer. Oncology, 71(1-2):18-25.

25. Ladas EJ (2014). Nutritional counseling in survivors of childhood cancer: An essential component of survivorship care. Children (Basel), 1(2):107-118.

26. Lang MJ, David V, and Giese-Davis J (2015). The age conundrum: A scoping review of younger age or adolescent and young adult as a risk factor for clinical distress, depression, or anxiety in cancer. Journal of Adolescent and Young Adult Oncology, 4(4):157-173.

27. Marks LB, Bentzen SM, Deasy JO, Kong FM, Bradley JD, Vogelius IS, El Naqa I, Hubbs JL, Lebesque JV, Timmerman RD, Martel MK, and Jackson A (2010). Radiation dose volume effects in the lung. International Journal of Radiation Oncology, Biology, and Physics, 76:S70-S76.

28. McDonnell G, Baily C, Schuler T, and Verdeli H (2015). Anxiety among adolescent survivors of pediatric cancer: A missing link in the survivorship literature. Palliative and Supportive Care, 13:345-349.

29. Melisko ME, Gradishar WJ, and Moy B (2016). Issues in breast cancer survivorship: Optimal care, bone health, and lifestyle modifications. American Society of Clinical Oncology Educational Book, 35:e22-e29.

30. Mell LK, Sirák I, Wei L, Tarnawski R, Mahantshetty U, Yashar CM, McHale MT, Xu R, Honerkamp-Smith G, Carmona R, Wright M, Williamson CW, Kasaová L, Li N, Kry S, Michalski J, Bosch W, Straube W, Schwarz J, Lowenstein J, Jiang SB, Saenz CC, Plaxe S, Einck J, Khorprasert C, Koonings P, Harrison T, Shi M, and Mundt AJ (2017). Bone marrow-sparing intensity modulated radiation therapy with concurrent cisplatin for stage ib-iva cervical cancer: An International Multicenter Phase II Clinical Trial (INTERTECC-2). International Journal of Radiation Oncology, Biology, and Physics, 97(3):536-545.

31. Milano MT, Li H, Gail MH, Constine LS, and Travis LB (2010). Long-term survival among patients with Hodgkin's lymphoma who developed breast cancer: A population-based study. Journal of Clinical Oncology, 28:5088-5096.

32. Milano MT, Strawderman RL, Venigalla S, Ng K, and Travis LB (2014). Non-small-cell lung cancer after breast cancer: A population-based study of clinicopathologic characteristics and survival outcomes in 3529 women. Journal Of Thoracic Oncology, 9(8):1081-1090.

33. Miller KD, Siegel RL, Lin CC, Mariotto AB, Kramer JL, Rowland JH, Stein KD, Alteri R, and Jemal A (2016). Cancer treatment and survivorship statistics, 2016. CA: A Cancer Journal for Clinicians, 66(4):271-289.

34. Mitchell AJ, Ferguson DW, Gill J, Paul J, and Symonds P (2013). Depression and anxiety in long-term cancer survivors compared with spouses and healthy controls: A systematic review and meta-analysis. The Lancet Oncology, 14(8):721-732.

35. Mustian KM, Sprod LK, Janelsins M, Peppone LJ, Palesh OG, Chandwani K, Reddy PS, Melnik MK, Heckler C, and Morrow GR (2013). Multicenter, randomized controlled trial of yoga for sleep quality among cancer survivors. Journal of Clinical Oncology, 31(26):3233-3241.

36. Mustian KM, Cole CL, Lin PJ, Asare M, Fung C, Janelsins M, Kamen C, Peppone L, and Magnuson A (2016). Exercise recommendations for the management of symptoms clusters resulting from cancer and cancer treatments. Seminars in Oncology Nursing, 32:383-393.

37. Nieman CL, Kazer R, Brannigan RE, Zoloth LS, Chase-Lansdale PL, Kinahan K, Dilley KJ, Roberts D, Shea LD, and Woodruff TK (2006). Cancer survivors and infertility: A review of a new problem and novel answers. Journal of Supportive Oncology, 4(4):171-178.

38. Pan HY, Haffty BG, Falit BP, Buchholz TA, Wilson LD, Hahn SM, and Smith BD (2016). Supply and demand for radiation oncology in the United States: Updated projections for 2015 to 2025. International Journal of Radiation Oncology, Biology, and Physics, 96(3):493-500.

39. Rim SH, Guy GP, Jr., Yabroff KR, McGraw KA, and Ekwueme DU (2016). The impact of chronic conditions on the economic burden of cancer survivorship: A systematic review. Expert Review of Pharmacoeconomics and Outcomes Research, 16(5):579-589.

40. Rock CL, Doyle C, Demark-Wahnefried W, Meyerhardt J, Courneya KS, Schwartz AL, Bandera EV, Hamilton KK, Grant B, McCullough M, Byers T, and Gansler T (2012). Nutrition and physical activity guidelines for cancer survivors. CA: A Cancer Journal for Clinicians, 62(4):243-274.

41. Runowicz CD, Leach CR, Henry NL, Henry KS, Mackey HT, Cowens-Alvarado RL, Cannady RS, Pratt-Chapman ML, Edge SB, Jacobs LA, Hurria A, Marks LB, LaMonte SJ, Warner E, Lyman GH, and Ganz PA (2016). American Cancer Society/American Society of Clinical Oncology Breast Cancer Survivorship Care Guideline. Journal of Clinical Oncology, 34(6):611-635.

42. Runowicz CD, Leach CR, Henry NL, Henry KS, Mackey HT, Cowens-Alvarado RL, Cannady RS, Pratt-Chapman ML, Edge SB, Jacobs LA, Hurria A, Marks LB, LaMonte SJ, Warner E, Lyman GH, and Ganz PA (2016). American Cancer Society/American Society of Clinical Oncology Breast Cancer Survivorship Care Guideline. CA: A Cancer Journal for Clinicians, 66(1):43-73.

43. Saphner T, Tormey DC, and Gray R (1991). Venous and arterial thrombosis in patients who received adjuvant therapy for breast cancer. Journal of Clinical Oncology, 9(2):286-294.

44. Sardar P, Kundu A, Chatterjee S, Nohria A, Nairooz R, Bangalore S, Mukherjee D, Aronow WS, and Lavie CJ (2017). Long-term cardiovascular mortality after radiotherapy for breast cancer: A systematic review and meta-analysis. Clinical Cardiology, 40(2):73-81.

45. Schneider BP, Hershman DL, and Loprinzi C (2015). Symptoms: Chemotherapy-induced peripheral neuropathy. Advances in Experimental Medicine and Biology, 862:77-87.

46. Smith RE, Bryant J, DeCillis A, Anderson S, National Surgical Adjuvant B, Bowel Project E (2003). Acute myeloid leukemia and myelodysplastic syndrome after doxorubicin-cyclophosphamide adjuvant therapy for operable breast cancer: The National Surgical Adjuvant Breast and Bowel Project Experience. Journal of Clinical Oncology, 21(7):1195-1204.

47. Staff NP, Grisold A, Grisold W, and Windebank AJ (2017). Chemotherapy-induced peripheral neuropathy: A current review. Annals of Neurology, 81(6):772-781.

48. Swartz MC, Lewis ZH, Lyons EJ, Jennings K, Middleton A, Deer RR, Arnold D, Dresser K, Ottenbacher KJ, and Goodwin JS (2017). Effect of home- and community-based physical activity interventions on physical function among cancer survivors: A systematic review and meta-analysis. Archives of Physical Medicine and Rehabilitation, 98(8):1652-1665.

49. Taylor C, Correa C, Duane FK, Aznar MC, Anderson SJ, Bergh J, Dodwell D, Ewertz M, Gray R, Jagsi R, Pierce L, Pritchard KI, Swain S, Wang Z, Wang Y, Whelan T, Peto R, and McGale P; Early Breast Cancer Trialists' Collaborative Group (2017). Estimating the risks of breast cancer radiotherapy: Evidence from modern radiation doses to the lungs and heart and from previous randomized trials. Journal of Clinical Oncology, 35(15):1641-1649.

50. Travis LB, Boice JD, Allan JM, Applegate KE, Constine LS, Gilbert ES, Kennedy AR, Ka-Min Ng A, Pui CH, Purdy JA, Xu Xg, and Yahalom J (2011). Report No. 170 - Second Primary Cancers and Cardiovascular Disease After Radiation Therapy. Bethesda: NCRP Publications.

51. Zhang FF, Kelly MJ, and Must A (2017). Early nutrition and physical activity interventions in childhood cancer survivors. Current Obesity Reports, 6(2):168-177.

52. Zhou ES, Nekhlyudov L, and Bober SL (2015). The primary health care physician and the cancer patient: tips and strategies for managing sexual health. Translational Andrology and Urology, 4(2):218-231.

BREAST CANCER AND THE PARTNER

Lidia Schapira, M.D., F.A.S.C.O.

INTRODUCTION

Receiving a diagnosis of breast cancer is a life-altering experience for any woman and her loved ones. A great deal of information and media attention have surrounded the topic of breast cancer, so it no longer is discussed in hushed tones. However, breast cancer is still experienced as deeply personal because the illness affects an organ typically associated with sexual intimacy, fertility, and motherhood.

Breast cancer affects not only a patient and her spouse or significant other (male and female spouses/significant others are hereafter referred to collectively as "partners," wherever appropriate), but also the rest of the inner family circle. In addition to other effects, the diagnosis and its treatment disrupt family routines. Women need their partners to be strong allies and advocates as they make important decisions and endure what can be grueling treatment regimens. They also need their partners to provide respite during this time from caregiving roles that they usually fulfill.

Both male and female partners may be thrown into roles that are unfamiliar, such as being the managing parent and principal caregiver in a household that may include children and/or aging parents. Cancer may even test the solidity of the union itself, as partners acclimate to new routines and roles and re-evaluate their intimate relationship. The partners also must work to ensure that they respect each other's point of view and negotiate workable compromises when it comes to decisions about treatment or family matters.

Open communication is key to maintaining normalcy during a period that is experienced as chaotic and frightening. I asked Marc Silver, author of *Breast Cancer Husband*, what he learned from the experience. He told me:

"We were in this together. I hope she drew strength from me (with my jokes and my back rubs) and I certainly drew strength from her fortitude and determination to get through the very difficult treatments. We say, 'I love you' to each other a lot more than before, because we have together faced this very difficult disease and

learned how wonderful it is to have each other."

BREAST CANCER AND SEXUAL INTIMACY

Surgery is an integral component of breast cancer treatment for many women and, for the majority, it is the first step in a multifaceted treatment plan. This is the first important treatment decision that a woman must make, one that will affect her body image, self-esteem, and psychological wellbeing. The degree to which partners participate in making these important decisions varies considerably. Partners tend to want information and to be included in decision-making, especially when treatment involves a mastectomy and different options for reconstruction. How each couple negotiates the role that partners play in this first step after diagnosis depends entirely on their relationship and style of communication. Surgeons can help by asking their patients if they wish to have their partners participate in decision-making and, if so, by respecting the partner's need to be informed and to participate in these important decisions.

Rowland and colleagues examined 17 studies that addressed men's experiences of their partner's body image following mastectomy and reconstructive surgery for treatment of breast cancer or for prophylaxis after genetic testing indicated a high risk of breast cancer. These researchers found that younger men were more affected than older men, that men did not like witnessing their partner in distress or pain from procedures, and that they experienced a period of mourning the loss of their partners' breast following mastectomy (Rowland, 2014). Although female partners of women with breast cancer were not included in this study, the feelings described are not gender-specific.

The literature reviewed by Rowland and colleagues also showed that women sometimes hid their naked bodies following their operations and that some husbands preferred not to look. Men described shifts in the level of intimacy and mourned the loss of their sexual intimacy. Men who were able to talk with their partners found that engaging in open communication helped them to come to terms with the diagnosis and trajectory of cancer, and this process led to reciprocal emotional support. These men said they did not talk to others about their wives' reconstruction and wished to share the responsibility of choosing the surgical procedure and type of reconstruction (Rowland, 2014). Again, these findings do not apply only to male partners.

The literature suggests that couples who see the cancer journey as a collaborative one and work together as a team to face the situation as a "we" may be better prepared to cope with the disruption and uncertainty associated with a cancer diagnosis (Thomas, 2002, and Kayser, 2007).

IMPACT OF TREATMENT ON PATIENTS' SELF-IMAGE

The physical changes that result from the partial or total removal of the breast have profound effects on the woman's body image, and other anti-cancer strategies have similar consequences. For example, radiation causes changes in skin color and the consistency of breast tissue and may restrict movement of the chest wall and upper arm. Systemic chemotherapy is difficult to endure, and side effects such as nausea are common. Premenopausal women typically experience a temporary cessation of menses during chemotherapy. Women in their 30s and early 40s may have menopausal symptoms such as hot flashes and joint stiffness, which usually subside in the months after chemotherapy ends. Women in the mid- to late-40s may experience amenorrhea that does not subside and may, in fact, transition into menopause; the associated decrease in available estrogen also may result in vaginal dryness as well as a significant decrease in libido.

Women of all ages with endocrine-sensitive breast cancer are now treated with longer courses of adjuvant endocrine therapy. For example, younger women now are treated with tamoxifen for up to 10 years, based on the results of large, randomized trials that showed a prolonged beneficial effect from a longer duration of therapy (Davies, 2013). Although controversy remains regarding the role of ovarian suppressive therapy for premenopausal women with estrogen-receptor—positive breast cancer, the results of a global randomized clinical trial showed that patients younger than 35 years of age at diagnosis with high-risk disease that warranted the use of adjuvant chemotherapy may benefit from ovarian suppression combined with either tamoxifen or aromatase inhibitors (Francis, 2014). All of these interventions, especially the use of ovarian suppressive therapy and aromatase inhibitors, cause vaginal atrophy and contribute to dyspareunia. Talking about these side effects may be difficult for a woman who struggles to reconcile her desire to "live" and adhere to medical treatment with complex feelings of body disfigurement and loss of function. Although couples together experience a sense of loss with changes in intimacy, it is often the partners who are more distressed, and these emotional struggles may go undetected or unexamined unless the topic is brought up by clinicians. Patients who are not asked about sexual intimacy may not volunteer this information, either because they feel they should be grateful for surviving and have no basis for "complaining," or that the clinician may not be able to provide any useful solutions for such problems.

HUSBANDS/MALE PARTNERS IN CAREGIVER ROLES

Stereotypical roles have men (and physicians, regardless of gender) in "fixing" roles. Research shows that many men invoke a gender-specific type of caregiving, characterized by many of the features typically associated with masculinity, including machoism, strength, rationality, courage, and instrumentality (Gilbert, 2002). For women, the term "caregiving" generally implies being supportive, emotionally available, nurturing, and flexible. As a result, men may not have much experience fulfilling their partner's expectations of caregiving and find this view of the role challenging and unintuitive.

I asked Marc Silver to comment on his experience and research of husbands as caregivers. He said:

"We're supposed to be the protectors of our family. When my wife was diagnosed with breast cancer, I thought my job should be to find the best docs and treatment plans for her. I learned from experience that being a cancer caregiver means, first of all, understanding that the cancer patient is the boss, and that your job as a caregiver is to support her throughout the difficult months of diagnosis and treatment. That you can tell her what you think but that she will make the decisions about her medical care. And that you need to figure out what she needs to get through it all."

High levels of self-silencing also have been found in male cancer caregivers, manifested as the propensity to engage in compulsive caretaking, pleasing others, and inhibition of self-expression in relationships in an attempt to achieve intimacy and meet relational needs (Gilbert, 2014). This "sturdy oak" masculine identity position was found to be co-constructed within heterosexual couples facing cancer, with women partners expressing emotion and allowing men to be stoic and strong (Seymour-Smith, 2006).

Silver adds: *"You have to learn to listen to your wife rather than be a cheerleader. Someone said to me that breast cancer husbands have to "shut up and listen." This means letting go of your idea of what should be done and really sitting back and listening to your wife. Sounds easy, turns out to be tough for a lot of guys."*

PARENTING

Approximately 20% of women with breast cancer have children under 18 at home; as a consequence, approximately 65,000 children in the United States are affected by this disease every year (Lewis, 2014). Predictably, studies show that children are negatively affected: school-age children may show regression, withdrawal, and anxiety about the stability of the family, and may worry their mother will die. An estimated 22% to 33% of children reach clinical levels of distress (Lewis, 2014). Mothers have reported that their own anxiety and worries kept them from being responsive to their child, saying they were in "survival mode," and not knowing how or if they should talk about their own worries with their children (Rauch, 2004, and Lewis, 2014). When parents do talk to their children about a mother's breast cancer diagnosis, many focus on technical or medical aspects instead of eliciting, listening to, and responding to their children's concerns.

Children may hold back on showing their distress or asking questions and may hide their thoughts and feelings so as not to upset their parents. One 9-year-old girl reported, "I went on the couch in front of the TV so she'd think that I'd been watching it, but I closed my eyes and I was thinking about her illness" (Lewis, 2014). Child life specialists and mental health professionals with pediatric training can help parents understand their children's concerns by focusing on the child's developmental stage, his or her temperament, and the family's communication style and beliefs. What is most important is to listen to the child's questions and to draw out their deepest fears and concerns. Many children ask if their mother will lose a breast, her hair, and her life, and parents need to be prepared to respond.

Teenagers, who may not be forthcoming about their feelings or may hide their emotions more capably, also are deeply affected. Adolescents may feel especially uncertain if they feel their parents are withholding information. Typically, adolescence is a time for "me first," so teens may be conflicted about their desire to separate from family and, at the same time, their desire to be around and supportive. Teens may be asked to take on adult roles in the household and care for younger siblings or prepare meals, but it is important also to allow them to have some time for friends and fun. Maintaining open lines of communication is key, and this can be accomplished creatively by exchanging notes, texting, or emailing—methods that may feel more comfortable than face-to-face discussions for adolescents struggling to accommodate their mixed emotions. Breast cancer may cause parents to shift roles, and this will likely affect the family dynamics providing many opportunities for both closeness and conflict.

COPING

Couples who are mutually attentive, recognize the needs of the other, and who openly communicate are more able to engage in effective coping styles, leading to positive experiences such as increased relationship closeness (Gilbert, 2014).

Marc Silver shared this important insight, based on his own experience:

"The hardest was ...coping with the uncertainty of diagnosis, before all the facts were in, was difficult. How serious was this cancer? What was Marsha's prognosis? These questions preyed on my mind. I felt as if my world, our world, was falling apart. I didn't know if I would have the strength to cope. And little by little, I learned that humans are pretty strong. That even if you've never been tested before, you can still be strong and carry on."

Partners of patients with breast cancer experience distress in amounts equal to that of patients and, in many cases, actually experience greater distress. Research on husbands/male partners has shown that, compared to the general population, these partners of women with breast cancer report lower quality of life and higher levels of depression and anxiety, as well as feelings of helplessness, exhaustion and fear (Brandao, 2014). It is reasonable to assume that these consequences also affect female partners of women with breast cancer.

> *To date, research on how partners cope with breast cancer and the impact of both disease and treatment on sexual function have focused on heterosexual couples. Less is known about sexual problems in women who identify as lesbian or bisexual, a group identified as a sexual minority in the medical literature. Women with female partners may encounter institutional and social barriers that prevent them from using some of the supportive resources available to heterosexual women, or they may feel uncomfortable in support groups designed for heterosexual couples (Paul, 2014). To be supportive of all patients, clinicians must acknowledge these potential barriers and should investigate and discuss what interventions or resources may help each particular couple or partner to cope with the illness on a case-by-case basis.*

HOW CLINICIANS CAN HELP

Clinicians can help both male and female partners of patients with cancer by "checking-in" with a simple, "How is this going for you?" or "Are you holding up okay?" Physicians and nurses can praise caregiving partners for their effort and dedication, offer caregiving tips and reassurance, and assign tasks to confirm their vital roles in the team effort. Very importantly, clinicians must recognize the partner's important role and provide guidance if he or she appears to be faltering.

Clinicians need to remember that partners appreciate clear and straightforward explanations of what is going on, and that they are moved and comforted by expressions of sympathy when diagnostic tests turn up bad news.

Marc Silver shared an anecdote that illustrates this point:

"Boy, you guys just can't catch a break," said my wife's surgeon when it appeared Marsha also had lymphoma in addition to breast cancer. Fortunately, she did not, as it turned out. But that simple and human expression of empathy made us feel better. "

In addition, psychological interventions can benefit both partners. Four important elements are common to any effective intervention: 1) a significant psychoeducational component designed to provide information about the cancer and normalize responses; 2) promotion of emotional expression and social support; 3) addressing sexual and body adaptation; and 4) focusing on finding some benefit in the experience and meaning in life (Brandao, 2014).

CONCLUSION

Partners of women with breast cancer are affected by the disease and experience significant degrees of emotional distress. Breast cancer may disrupt family routines and cause shifts in relationships and roles, leaving partners to assume greater responsibilities as caregivers. Couples who see the cancer journey as a collaborative one and work together as a team are better prepared to cope with the disruption and uncertainty associated with a cancer diagnosis. Clinicians must recognize the impact of the disease on the patient's spouse/partner and on the relationship itself as a first step, and then offer guidance and support.

REFERENCES

1. Davies C, Pan H, Godwin J, Gray R, Arriagada R, Raina V, Abraham M, Medeiros Alencar VH, Badran A, Bonfill X, Bradbury J, Clarke M, Collins R, Davis SR, Delmestri A, Forbes JF, Haddad P, Hou MF, Inbar M, Khaled H, Kielanowska J, Kwan WH, Mathew BS, Mittra I, Müller B, Nicolucci A, Peralta O, Pernas F, Petruzelka L, Pienkowski T, Radhika R, Rajan B, Rubach MT, Tort S, Urrútia G, Valentini M, Wang Y, and Peto R; Adjuvant Tamoxifen: Longer Against Shorter (ATLAS) Collaborative Group (2013). Long-term effects of continuing adjuvant tamoxifen to 10 years versus stopping at 5 years after diagnosis of oestrogen receptor-positive breast cancer: ATLAS, a randomised trial. Lancet, 381 (9869):805-816.

2. Francis PA, Regan MM, Fleming GF, Láng I, Ciruelos E, Bellet M, Bonnefoi HR, Climent MA, Da Prada GA, Burstein HJ, Martino S, Davidson NE, Geyer CE Jr, Walley BA, Coleman R, Kerbrat P, Buchholz S, Ingle JN, Winer EP, Rabaglio-Poretti M, Maibach R, Ruepp B, Giobbie-Hurder A, Price KN, Colleoni M, Viale G, Coates AS, Goldhirsch A, and Gelber RD; SOFT Investigators; International Breast Cancer Study Group (2015). Adjuvant ovarian suppression in premenopausal breast cancer. New England Journal of Medicine, 372(5):436-446.

3. Gilbert E, Ussher JM, and Perz J (2014). 'Not that I want to be thought of as a hero': Narrative analysis of performative masculinities and the experience of informal cancer caring. Psychology and Health, 29(12):1442-1457.

4. Kayser K, Watson LE, and Andrade JT (2007). Cancer as a "we disease": Examining the process of coping from a relational perspective. Families, Systems and Health, (25):404-418.

5. Lewis FM, Brandt PA, Cochrane BB, Griffith KA, Grant M, Haase JE, Houldin AD, Post-White J, Zahlis EH, and Shands ME (2014). The enhancing connections program: A six-state randomized clinical trial of a cancer parenting program. Journal of Consulting and Clinical Psychology, (83(1):12-23.

6. Maughan K, Heyman B, and Matthews M (2002). In the shadow of risk. How men cope with a partner's gynecological cancer. International Journal of Nursing Studies, 39(1):27-34.

7. Paul LB, Pitagora D, Brown B, Tworecke A, and Rubin L (2014). Support needs and resources of sexual minority women with breast cancer. Psycho-oncology, 23(5):578-584.

8. Rauch PK and Muriel AC (2004). The importance of parenting concerns among patients with cancer. Critical Reviews in Oncology/Hematology, 49(1):37-42.

9. Rowland E and Metcalfe A (2014). A systematic review of men's experiences of their partners' mastectomy: Coping with altered bodies. Psycho-oncology, 23(9):963-974.

10. Seymour-Smith S and Wetherell M (2006). 'What he hasn't told you...': Investigating the micro-politics of gendered support in heterosexual couples' co-constructed accounts of illness. Feminism and Psychology, 16(1):105-127.

11. Thomas C, Morris SM, and Harman JC (2002). Companions through cancer: The care given by informal carers in cancer contexts. Social Science and Medicine, 54(4):529-544.

RELATIONSHIPS BETWEEN COGNITIVE IMPAIRMENTS IN BREAST CANCER SURVIVORS AND MENOPAUSE

Allison M. Magnuson, D.O. and Michelle Janelsins, Ph.D., M.P.H.

CANCER-RELATED COGNITIVE IMPAIRMENT (CRCI)

Cancer-related cognitive impairment (CRCI), sometimes referred to as "chemobrain," is an important clinical problem for breast cancer survivors. Cancer-related cognitive impairment involves a set of commonly reported problems in memory, attention, concentration, processing, and executive function (Janelsins, 2011; Janelsins, 2014; and Ahles, 2017). Cancer-related cognitive impairment often is more subtle compared to many other central nervous system disorders or neurodegenerative diseases, yet it is debilitating and can begin prior to treatment, during treatment, and can linger for several years beyond treatment. Based on data from several types of cancers, up to 30% of survivors experience cognitive impairment prior to therapy, 80% during therapy, and up to 35% may experience CRCI up to 20 years after treatment (Koppelmans, 2012; Joly, 2015; Wefel, 2015; and Janelsins, 2016). Treatments related to CRCI include chemotherapy, which is the most studied, as well as radiation therapy and endocrine therapy. Some studies have provided evidence for CRCI prior to systemic therapies and have implicated surgery as a possible factor (Hedayati, 2011) as well as the finding that CRCI may exist prior to both surgery and chemotherapy (Hermelink, 2007). Cancer-related cognitive impairment has been most studied in breast cancer, which is where most of the evidence is derived, but CRCI is not specific to a breast cancer diagnosis alone. A growing body of literature also provides evidence for CRCI in colon, lymphoma, and prostate cancers as well (Ahles, 2002; Vardy, 2015; and Wu, 2016). Cancer-related cognitive impairment is associated with poorer quality of life, inability to achieve work and educational goals, problems with reading or driving, and decreased social connectivity. Cancer-related cognitive impairment also can interfere with the ability to live independently for some adults (Reid-Arndt, 2010, and Selamat, 2014).

FACTORS CONTRIBUTING TO CRCI

Many demographic, medical, biologic, psychologic, and other symptom factors could influence and contribute to CRCI in adults with breast cancer (Table 1).

Table 1: Possible Factors Related to Cancer-Related Cognitive Impairment in the Breast Cancer Survivor

Demographic/ Host Factors	Cancer-related Medical	Other Medical and Biologic Factors	Psychologic and Other Symptoms
Age	Disease stage and type	Menopausal status	Anxiety
Education	Surgery	Comorbid conditions	Depression
Race/Ethnicity	Chemotherapy	Inflammation and neuro-immune factors	Stress
Cognitive reserve	Radiation	Metabolic processes	Fatigue
	Hormone therapy	Genetic factors	Sleep disturbance

Demographic Factors

By 2020, it is estimated that two-thirds of all cancer survivors will be 65 years of age or older (Stouten-Kemperman, 2015). Cancer and its treatment may exacerbate normal aging processes and increase cognitive impairment in older breast cancer survivors (Mandelblatt, 2014, and Williams, 2015). The section below further details considerations for older adults. However, it is important to consider that both younger and older adults with breast cancer experience CRCI (Mandelblatt, 2014, and Janelsins, 2016). Cognitive reserve, assessed by the Wide Range Achievement Test (WRAT) Reading scale, has suggested that lower innate cognitive capacity (taking into account education, environment, and occupation) prior to chemotherapy treatments explains the risk for post-treatment decline in processing speed (Ahles, 2010). Other factors that may influence CRCI include education, race, and ethnicity (Mandelblatt, 2014, and Janelsins, 2016).

Medical Factors:
A Focus on Cancer Treatments and Menopausal Status

Several medical factors could impact CRCI including stage of disease, treatment types, comorbid conditions, and body mass index (Loef, 2012; Sherwin, 2012; and Loef, 2013). Most of the literature focuses on chemotherapy; however, recent studies have shed light on the impact of hormonal therapies for certain types of hormone receptor positive breast cancers and the impact of menopausal status. For example, post-treatment cognitive function and brain activation can vary by pre-treatment menopausal status (Conroy, 2013). Breast cancer patients who received chemotherapy and tamoxifen have been shown to have greater cognitive difficulties than those who received chemotherapy alone (Castellon, 2004). Another cross-sectional study assessing tamoxifen in pre-menopausal breast cancer patients compared to healthy controls found greater difficulty in visual and verbal memory and processing speed (Palmer, 2008). One prospective study found deterioration in verbal memory and executive function in post-menopausal patients taking tamoxifen for one year (but not in those taking the aromatase inhibitor (AI), exemestane, compared to healthy controls) (Schilder, 2010).

Hurria and colleagues evaluated cognition with neuropsychologic assessment in older women receiving AI therapy for adjuvant breast cancer treatment (Hurria, 2014). Women aged greater than or equal to 60 years were compared with age-matched controls at baseline and six months into treatment. They did not observe any significant decline in cognitive function in patients receiving AI therapy as compared to controls. Another study by Schilder and colleagues assessed the impact of tamoxifen and AI therapy on cognitive function in post-menopausal breast cancer patients (age 51 to 81) (Schilder, 2010). Women receiving tamoxifen performed worse than age-matched health controls in areas of verbal memory and executive function. No difference was observed in patients receiving AI therapy. Exploratory analysis on this study suggested that older patients (age greater than 65) receiving tamoxifen were most vulnerable to cognitive decline. Larger studies are needed to confirm these results and to address the combined effects of chemotherapy and endocrine therapy with menopausal status on cognitive function in cancer.

Biologic Factors

Peripheral blood markers representing the individual's specific physiologic status may help identify those at risk for CRCI. The most widely studied biomechanism related to CRCI has been inflammation; studies show that inflammation is associated with CRCI before, during, and after chemotherapy. Most of the evidence surrounding inflammation supports a role for the tumor necrosis factor–alpha (TNF-α) pathway

147

(Ganz, 2013; Patel, 2015; Lyon, 2016; and Williams, 2017). Increased inflammation could be related to CRCI directly or an indicator of other physiologic processes that are related to CRCI; further studies are needed to tease apart the role of inflammation on CRCI.

Genetic factors also have been investigated for their role in moderating or mediating effects of CRCI. Genes in lipid metabolism pathways (i.e., apolipoprotein E [APOE]) (Ahles, 2003), neurotransmitter signaling (catechol-O-methyltransferase [COMT]) (Small, 2011), and growth factor (brain derived neurotrophic factor [BDNF]) (Ng, 2016) all have been implicated in CRCI risk, although further confirmatory studies are needed.

Psychologic and Symptom Factors

Several psychologic and symptom sequelae may be related to CRCI including anxiety, depression, sleep disturbances, and fatigue. These factors often are highly correlated with subjective cognitive measures; however, the trajectories of changes in symptoms with changes in subjective and objective cognitive outcomes still are not well understood. Additional research is needed to understand how psychologic factors and symptoms—all of which correlate with but are distinct processes from CRCI—may moderate or mediate effects on cognitive performance (Morrow, 2005; Ryan, 2007; Vearncombe, 2009; Mustian, 2012; and Palesh, 2012). Fully understanding the impact of psychologic and symptom changes as they relate to those who have CRCI, particularly early on during treatment as well as persistent CRCI, will help aid in the development of interventions to alleviate CRCI and other related outcomes.

CONSIDERATIONS FOR OLDER ADULTS

Older adults represent the largest group of adult breast cancer survivors, and they pose a unique consideration when evaluating chemotherapy-related cognitive impairment, colloquially known as "chemo brain." Aging is a risk factor for cognitive impairment; however, the interplay between aging, cancer, and cancer therapy on cognition is not well understood. Additionally, there is concern that older adults with pre-existing changes in cognition may be more vulnerable to progressive cognitive decline with exposure to cancer therapies. Although there is increasing data regarding the effects of cancer and cancer treatment on cognition, the majority of this research has been

148

conducted in younger adults.

A few studies have evaluated self-reported change in memory in older adults receiving chemotherapy. One study evaluated subjective change in cognition with receipt of adjuvant chemotherapy for breast cancer (Hurria, 2006). Forty-five women aged 65 and older were evaluated with standardized questionnaires about their cognition (Squire Memory Self-rating Questionnaire) prior to receipt of chemotherapy and six months post treatment. Fifty-one percent of patients experienced subjective decline in their memory following chemotherapy, and this was most noticeable in patients who expressed concerns about their memory at baseline. However, another study evaluating self-reported cognitive function in older women receiving adjuvant chemotherapy for breast cancer did not find this (Freedman, 2013). In this study, self-reported cognitive function was assessed in 297 women aged greater than or equal to 65 who were enrolled in the quality of life sub study of the Cancer and Leukemia Group B (CALBG) 49907 study evaluating outcomes of adjuvant chemotherapy in breast cancer. Cognitive function was assessed with the Memory, Cognitive, and Concentration subscales of the Neurobehavioral Functioning and Activities of Daily Living scale at six time points around adjuvant chemotherapy receipt (baseline to 24 months post treatment). Investigators did not observe longitudinal changes in self-reported cognitive function in this group. In general, the population of patients enrolled in this study appeared to be more fit with less baseline concerns about memory as compared to those enrolled in the Hurria study. Additionally, different measures of memory self-rating were used in the two studies, which also may contribute to the discordant results.

Other studies have evaluated cognitive change using objective cognitive measures. In one such study, Lange and colleagues evaluated the impact of chemotherapy on cognition in women aged greater than or equal to 65 receiving adjuvant treatment for breast cancer using comprehensive neuropsychologic assessment before and after chemotherapy receipt (Lange, 2014). Investigators evaluated patients receiving either adjuvant chemotherapy (n=58) or adjuvant radiation therapy (n=61) and compared results to age-matched controls (n=62). They observed that 49% of patients receiving adjuvant treatment (either chemotherapy or radiation therapy) had objective cognitive decline following treatment, mainly in the area of working memory. The subgroup of older patients in the study (70+) tended to have more significant decline as compared to younger patients (65 to 69). In another smaller study of women receiving adjuvant therapy for breast cancer (n=28), neuropsychologic assessment was performed in patients pre- and post-receipt of chemotherapy (Hurria, 2006). In this study, 39% of patients experienced a decline in cognitive function following treatment. Interestingly, 11% of patients were noted to have improvement in cognition following therapy in this study. Another objective study of chemotherapy on cognition in adjuvant breast cancer by Ahles and colleagues included a subset of older patients (age greater than 60) and compared results to a younger adjuvant breast cancer population as well as to age-matched controls (Ahles, 2010). They observed that older patients who had lower cognitive reserve at baseline experienced the most significant decline after exposure to chemotherapy. There is limited data about the longer-term effects of cancer therapy on cognition in older adults. Mandelblatt and colleagues evaluated the late effects of cancer therapy on self-reported cognition in older breast cancer survivors (age 65 to 91, median 4.1 years after treatment) (Mandelblatt, 2016). They observed three patterns of cognitive change in this group of survivors over time. In 42.3% of patients, self-reported cognitive function was "maintained high," 50.1% of patients experienced "phase shift" with cognitive scores slightly below normal but with parallel decline over time as compared to the "maintained high" group, whereas 7.6% of patients experienced "accelerated decline" of cognition. Patients who received chemotherapy were 2.1 times more likely to experience accelerated decline, as compared to patients receiving endocrine therapy alone. This group of patients also was more likely to develop greater comorbidity and frailty.

MANAGEMENT OF CRCI AND CLINICAL IMPLICATIONS

Accurate clinical evaluation and description of cognitive impairments is important, because cognitive impairment can lead to poor treatment compliance, decreased quality of life, and interfere with the ability to work (Reid-Arndt, 2010, and Myers, 2012). Related to compliance, 80% of patients with chronic illness including cancer said they would not have chosen a treatment if they had known it would affect their cognitive ability (Fried, 2002), and cancer survivors who self-report cognitive difficulties have reported a negative impact on their quality of life (Schagen, 2008). Thus, concerns about cognitive problems should be evaluated and addressed by the treating physician, as well as psychologists and neurologists. Three measures recommended by the International Cancer and Cognition Task Force include the Hopkins Verbal Learning and Memory Test-Revised, the Controlled Oral Word Association Test, and the Trail Making Test. These could be utilized by clinicians and researchers to assess individual time-points or evaluate changes over time from prior to treatment into survivorship. Referrals to social workers and neuropsychologists also may be needed.

Physicians also may consider addressing psychologic concerns including anxiety, depression, and fatigue, as well as stressors, and may suggest coping strategies for managing cognitive complaints. Cognitive impairment is one of many adverse events that cancer survivors experience; increased physician and patient awareness of treatment history and the possible associated risks described herein will help to identify patients with CRCI and provide individualized care (Robison, 2014).

While researchers and clinicians are continuing to understand and characterize CRCI, efforts have begun to develop and test interventions that might alleviate or prevent CRCI in adults with breast cancer, although confirmatory trials on several promising interventions still are needed. Cognitive rehabilitation approaches that involve training to improve specific processes involved in CRCI, as well as management approaches to compensate for deficits, have both shown to be beneficial. These include in-person, one-on-one approaches with a therapist, group intervention sessions, and computerized training programs. Additional studies also suggest that physical activity interventions including yoga, qigong, tai chi, and walking programs may help alleviate memory difficulties and other aspects of CRCI. Lastly, while no pharmacologic intervention has been approved specifically for CRCI, some pharmacologic treatments also may be helpful. Studies suggest that modafinil and methylphenidate may provide benefit (Mar Fan, 2008; Kohli, 2009; Lundorff, 2009; Ferguson, 2012; Oh, 2012; Reid-Arndt, 2012; Sprod, 2012; Von Ah, 2012; Barton, 2013; and Kesler, 2013).

REFERENCES

1. Ahles TA, Saykin AJ, Furstenberg CT, Cole B, Mott LA, Skalla K, Whedon MB, Bivens S, Mitchell T, Greenberg ER, and Silberfarb PM (2002).. Neuropsychologic impact of standard-dose systemic chemotherapy in long-term survivors of breast cancer and lymphoma. Journal of

Clinical Oncology, 20(2):485-493

2. Ahles TA, Saykin AJ, Noll WW, Furstenberg CT, Guerin S, Cole B, ands Mott LA (2003). The relationship of APOE genotype to neuropsychological performance in long-term cancer survivors treated with standard dose chemotherapy. Psychooncology, 12(6):612-619.

3. Ahles TA, Saykin AJ, McDonald BC, Li Y, Furstenberg CT, Hanscom BS, Mulrooney TJ, Schwartz GN, and Kaufman PA (2010). Longitudinal assessment of cognitive changes associated with adjuvant treatment for breast cancer: Impact of age and cognitive reserve. Journal of Clinical Oncology, 28(29):4434-4440.

4. Ahles TA, and Root JC (2017). Cognitive Effects of Cancer and Cancer Treatments. Annual Review of Clinical Psychology, In Press.

5. Barton DL, Burger K, Novotny PJ, Fitch TR, Kohli S, Soori G, Wilwerding MB, Sloan JA, Kottschade LA, Rowland KM Jr, Dakhil SR, Nikcevich DA, and Loprinzi CL (2013). The use of Ginkgo biloba for the prevention of chemotherapy-related cognitive dysfunction in women receiving adjuvant treatment for breast cancer, N00C9. Support Care Cancer, 21(4):1185-1192.

6. Castellon SA, Ganz PA, Bower JE, Petersen L, Abraham L, and Greendale GA (2004). Neurocognitive performance in breast cancer survivors exposed to adjuvant chemotherapy and tamoxifen. Journal of Clinical and Exp Neuropsychol. 2004;26(7):955-969.

7. Conroy SK, McDonald BC, Ahles TA, West JD, and Saykin AJ (2013). Chemotherapy-induced amenorrhea: A prospective study of brain activation changes and neurocognitive correlates. Brain Imaging and Behavior, 7(4):491-500.

8. Ferguson RJ, McDonald BC, Rocque MA, Furstenberg CT, Horrigan S, Ahles TA, and Saykin AJ (2012). Development of CBT for chemotherapy-related cognitive change: Results of a waitlist control trial. Psychooncology, 21(2):176-186.

9. Freedman RA, Pitcher B, Keating NL, Ballman KV, Mandelblatt J, Kornblith AB, Kimmick GG, Hurria A, Winer EP, Hudis CA, Cohen HJ, and Muss HB (2013). Cognitive function in older women with breast cancer treated with standard chemotherapy and capecitabine on Cancer and Leukemia Group B 49907. Breast Cancer Research and Treatment, 139(2):607-616.

10. Fried TR, Bradley EH, Towle VR, and Allore H (2002). Understanding the treatment preferences of seriously ill patients. The New England Journal of Medicine, 346(14):1061-1066.

11. Ganz PA, Bower JE, Kwan L, Castellon SA, Silverman DH, Geist C, Breen EC, Irwin MR, and Cole SW (2013). Does tumor necrosis factor-alpha (TNF-alpha) play a role in post-chemotherapy cerebral dysfunction? Brain, Behavior, and Immunity, 30 Suppl:S99-108.

12. Hedayati E, Schedin A, Nyman H, Alinaghizadeh H, and Albertsson M (2011). The effects of breast cancer diagnosis and surgery on cognitive functions. Acta Oncologica, 50(7):1027-1036.

13. Hermelink K, Untch M, Lux MP, Kreienberg R, Beck T, Bauerfeind I, and Münzel K (2007). Cognitive function during neoadjuvant chemotherapy for breast cancer: Results of a prospective, multicenter, longitudinal study. Cancer, 109(9):1905-1913.

14. Hurria A, Rosen C, Hudis C, Zuckerman E, Panageas KS, Lachs MS, Witmer M, van Gorp WG, Fornier M, D'Andrea G, Moasser M, Dang C, Van Poznak C, Hurria A, and Holland J (2006).

Cognitive function of older patients receiving adjuvant chemotherapy for breast cancer: A pilot prospective longitudinal study. Journal of the American Geriatrics Society, 54(6):925-931.

15. Hurria A, Goldfarb S, Rosen C, Holland J, Zuckerman E, Lachs MS, Witmer M, van Gorp WG, Fornier M, D'Andrea G, Moasser M, Dang C, Van Poznak C, Robson M, Currie VE, Theodoulou M, Norton L, and Hudis C (2006). Effect of adjuvant breast cancer chemotherapy on cognitive function from the older patient's perspective. Breast Cancer Research and Treatment, 98(3):343-348.

16. Hurria A, Patel SK, Mortimer J, Luu T, Somlo G, Katheria V, Ramani R, Hansen K, Feng T, Chuang C, Geist CL, and Silverman DH (2014). The effect of aromatase inhibition on the cognitive function of older patients with breast cancer. Clinical Breast Cancer, 14(2):132-140.

17. Janelsins MC, Kohli S, Mohile SG, Usuki K, Ahles TA, and Morrow GR (2011). An update on cancer- and chemotherapy-related cognitive dysfunction: Current status. Seminars in Oncology, 38(3):431-438.

18. Janelsins MC, Kesler SR, Ahles TA, and Morrow GR (2014). Prevalence, mechanisms, and management of cancer-related cognitive impairment. International Review of Psychiatry, 26(1):102-113.

19. Janelsins MC, Heckler CE, Peppone LJ, Kamen C, Mustian KM, Mohile SG, Magnuson A, Kleckner IR, Guido JJ, Young KL, Conlin AK, Weiselberg LR, Mitchell JW, Ambrosone CA, Ahles TA, and Morrow GR (2016). Cognitive complaints in survivors of breast cancer after chemotherapy compared with age-matched controls: An analysis from a nationwide, multicenter, prospective longitudinal study. Journal of clinical oncology: Official journal of the American Society of Clinical Oncology. 35(5):506-514.

20. Joly F, Giffard B, Rigal O, De Ruiter MB, Small BJ, Dubois M, LeFel J, Schagen SB, Ahles TA, Wefel JS, Vardy JL, Pancré V, Lange M, and Castel H (2015). Impact of cancer and its treatments on cognitive function: advances in research from the paris international cognition and cancer task force symposium and update since 2012. Journal of Pain and Symptom Management, 50(6):830-841.

21. Kesler S, Hadi Hosseini SM, Heckler C, Janelsins M, Palesh O, Mustian K, and Morrow G (2013). Cognitive training for improving executive function in chemotherapy-treated breast cancer survivors. Clinical Breast Cancer, 13(4):299-306.

22. Kohli S, Fisher SG, Tra Y, Adams MJ, Mapstone ME, Wesnes KA, Roscoe JA, and Morrow GR (2009). The effect of modafinil on cognitive function in breast cancer survivors. Cancer, 115(12):2605-2616.

23. Koppelmans V, Breteler MM, Boogerd W, Seynaeve C, Gundy C, and Schagen SB (2012). Neuropsychological performance in survivors of breast cancer more than 20 years after adjuvant chemotherapy. Journal of Clinical Oncology, 30(10):1080-1086.

24. Lange M, Giffard B, Noal S, Rigal O, Kurtz JE, Heutte N, Lévy C, Allouache D, Rieux C, Le Fel J, Daireaux A, Clarisse B, Veyret C, Barthélémy P, Longato N, Eustache F, and Joly F (2014).

Baseline cognitive functions among elderly patients with localised breast cancer. European Journal of Cancer, 50(13):2181-2189.

25. Loef M and Walach H (2012). Fruit, vegetables and prevention of cognitive decline or dementia: A systematic review of cohort studies. Journal of Nutrition, Health, and Aging, 16(7):626-630.

26. Loef M and Walach H (2013). Midlife obesity and dementia: Meta-analysis and adjusted forecast of dementia prevalence in the United States and China. Obesity, 21(1):E51-55.

27. Lundorff LE, Jonsson BH, and Sjogren P (2009). Modafinil for attentional and psychomotor dysfunction in advanced cancer: A double-blind, randomised, cross-over trial. Palliative Medicine, 23(8):731-738.

28. Lyon DE, Cohen R, Chen H, Kelly DL, McCain NL, Starkweather A, Ahn H, Sturgill J, and Jackson-Cook CK (2016). Relationship of systemic cytokine concentrations to cognitive function over two years in women with early stage breast cancer. Journal of Neuroimmunology, 301:74-82.

29. Mandelblatt JS, Jacobsen PB, and Ahles T (2014) Cognitive effects of cancer systemic therapy: Implications for the care of older patients and survivors. Journal of Clinical Oncology, 32(24):2617-2626.

30. Mandelblatt JS, Clapp JD, Luta G, Faul LA, Tallarico MD, McClendon TD, Whitley JA, Cai L, Ahles TA, Stern RA, Jacobsen PB, Small BJ, Pitcher BN, Dura-Fernandis E, Muss HB, Hurria A, Cohen HJ, and Isaacs C (2016). Long-term trajectories of self-reported cognitive function in a cohort of older survivors of breast cancer: CALGB 369901 (Alliance). Cancer, 122:3555-3563.

31. Mar Fan HG, Clemons M, Xu W, Chemerynsky I, Breunis H, Braganza S, and Tannock IF (2008). A randomised, placebo-controlled, double-blind trial of the effects of d-methylphenidate on fatigue and cognitive dysfunction in women undergoing adjuvant chemotherapy for breast cancer. Support Care Cancer, 16(6):577-583.

32. Morrow GR, Shelke AR, Roscoe JA, Hickok JT, and Mustian K (2005). Management of cancer-related fatigue. Cancer Investigation, 23(3):229-239.

33. Mustian KM, Sprod LK, Janelsins M, Peppone LJ, and Mohile S (2012). Exercise recommendations for cancer-related fatigue, cognitive impairment, sleep problems, depression, pain, anxiety, and physical dysfunction: A review. Oncology and Hematology Review, 8(2):81-88.

34. Myers JS (2012). Chemotherapy-related cognitive impairment: The breast cancer experience. Oncology Nursing Forum, 39(1):E31-40.

35. Ng T, Teo SM, Yeo HL, Shwe M, Gan YX, Cheung YT, Foo KM, Cham MT, Lee JA, Tan YP, Fan G, Yong WS, Preetha M, Loh WJ, Koo SL, Jain A, Lee GE, Wong M, Dent R, Yap YS, Ng R, Khor CC, Ho HK, and Chan A (2016). Brain-derived neurotrophic factor genetic polymorphism (rs6265) is protective against chemotherapy-associated cognitive impairment in patients with early-stage breast cancer. Neuro-Oncology, 18(2):244-251.

36. Oh B, Butow PN, Mullan BA, Clarke SJ, Beale PJ, Pavlakis N, Lee MS, Rosenthal DS, Larkey L, and Vardy J (2012). Effect of medical Qigong on cognitive function, quality of life, and a

biomarker of inflammation in cancer patients: A randomized controlled trial. Support Care in Cancer, 20(6):1235-1242.

37. Palesh O, Peppone L, Innominato PF, Janelsins M, Jeong M, Sprod L, Savard J, Rotatori M, Kesler S, Telli M, and Mustian K (2012). Prevalence, putative mechanisms, and current management of sleep problems during chemotherapy for cancer. Nat and Science of Sleep, 4:151-162.

38. Palmer JL, Trotter T, Joy AA, and Carlson LE (2008). Cognitive effects of Tamoxifen in pre-menopausal women with breast cancer compared to healthy controls. Journal of Cancer Survivorship, 2(4):275-282.

39. Patel SK, Wong AL, Wong FL, Breen EC, Hurria A, Smith M, Kinjo C, Paz IB, Kruper L, Somlo G, Mortimer JE, Palomares MR, Irwin MR, and Bhatia S (2015). Inflammatory biomarkers, comorbidity, and neurocognition in women with newly diagnosed breast cancer. Journal of the National Cancer Institute, 107(8).pii: djv131. doi: 10.1093/jnci/djv131.

40. Reid-Arndt SA, Hsieh C, and Perry MC (2010). Neuropsychological functioning and quality of life during the first year after completing chemotherapy for breast cancer. Psycho-oncology, 19(5):535-544.

41. Reid-Arndt SA, Matsuda S, and Cox CR (2012). Tai Chi effects on neuropsychological, emotional, and physical functioning following cancer treatment: A pilot study. Complementary Therapies in Clinical Practice, 18(1):26-30.

42. Robison LL and Hudson MM (2014). Survivors of childhood and adolescent cancer: Life-long risks and responsibilities. Nature reviews.Cancer. 14(1):61-70.

43. Ryan JL, Carroll JK, Ryan EP, Mustian KM, Fiscella K, and Morrow GR (2007). Mechanisms of cancer-related fatigue. Oncologist, 12 Suppl 1:22-34.

44. Selamat MH, Loh SY, Mackenzie L, and Vardy J (2014). Chemobrain experienced by breast cancer survivors: A meta-ethnography study investigating research and care implications. PLoS One, 9(9):e108002.

45. Schagen SB, Boogerd W, Muller MJ, Huinink WT, Moonen L, Meinhardt W, and Van Dam FS (2008). Cognitive complaints and cognitive impairment following BEP chemotherapy in patients with testicular cancer. Acta oncologica (Stockholm, Sweden). 47(1):63-70.Schilder CM, Seynaeve C, Beex LV, Boogerd W, Linn SC, Gundy CM, Huizenga HM, Nortier JW, van de Velde CJ, van Dam FS, and Schagen SB (2010). Effects of tamoxifen and exemestane on cognitive functioning of postmenopausal patients with breast cancer: Results from the neuropsychological side study of the tamoxifen and exemestane adjuvant multinational trial. Journal of Clinical Oncology, 28(8):1294-1300.

46. Sherwin BB (2012). Estrogen and cognitive functioning in women: Lessons we have learned. Behavioral Neuroscience, 126(1):123-127.

47. Small BJ, Rawson KS, Walsh E, Jim HS, Hughes TF, Iser L, Andrykowski MA, and Jacobsen PB (2011). Catechol-O-methyltransferase genotype modulates cancer treatment-related

cognitive deficits in breast cancer survivors. Cancer, 117(7):1369-1376.

48. Sprod LK, Mohile SG, Demark-Wahnefried W, Janelsins MC, Peppone LJ, Morrow GR, Lord R, Gross H, and Mustian KM (2012). Exercise and cancer treatment symptoms in 408 newly diagnosed older cancer patients. Journal of Geriatric Oncology, 3(2):90-97.

49. Stouten-Kemperman MM, de Ruiter MB, Koppelmans V, Boogerd W, Reneman L, and Schagen SB (2015). Neurotoxicity in breast cancer survivors >/=10 years post-treatment is dependent on treatment type. Brain Imaging and Behavior, 9(2):275-284.

50. Vardy JL, Dhillon HM, Pond GR, Rourke SB, Bekele T, Renton C, Dodd A, Zhang H, Beale P, Clarke S, and Tannock IF (2015). Cognitive function in patients with colorectal cancer who do and do not receive chemotherapy: A prospective, longitudinal, controlled study. Journal of Clinical Oncology, 33(34):4085-4092.

51. Vearncombe KJ, Rolfe M, Wright M, Pachana NA, Andrew B, and Beadle G (2009). Predictors of cognitive decline after chemotherapy in breast cancer patients. Journal of the International Neuropsychological Society, 15(6):951-962.

52. Von Ah D, Carpenter JS, Saykin A, Monahan P, Wu J, Yu M, Rebok G, Ball K, Schneider B, Weaver M, Tallman E, and Unverzagt F (2012). Advanced cognitive training for breast cancer survivors: A randomized controlled trial. Breast Cancer Research and Treatment, 135(3):799-809.

53. Wefel JS, Kesler SR, Noll KR, and Schagen SB (2015). Clinical characteristics, pathophysiology, and management of noncentral nervous system cancer-related cognitive impairment in adults. CA: A Cancer Journal for Clinicians, 65(2):123-138.

54. Williams AM, Janelsins MC, and van Wijngaarden E (2015). Cognitive function in cancer survivors: analysis of the 1999-2002 National Health and Nutrition Examination Survey. Supportive Care in Cancer, 24(5):2155-2162.

55. Williams AM, Shah R, Shayne M, Huston AJ, Krebs M, Murray N, Thompson BD, Doyle K, Korotkin J, van Wijngaarden E, Hyland S, Moynihan JA, Cory-Slechta DA, and Janelsins MC (2017). Associations between inflammatory markers and cognitive function in breast cancer patients receiving chemotherapy. Journal of neuroimmunology, S0165-5728(17)30198-30204.

56. Wu LM, Tanenbaum ML, Dijkers MP, Amidi A, Hall SJ, Penedo FJ, and Diefenbach MA (2016). Cognitive and neurobehavioral symptoms in patients with non-metastatic prostate cancer treated with androgen deprivation therapy or observation: A mixed methods study. Social Science and Medicine, 156:80-89.

THE BIOLOGY AND MANAGEMENT OF LYMPHEDEMA IN THE BREAST CANCER PATIENT

Jayne E. Knowlton, M.S., O.T.R./L.
and Shirley S. Mandeville, F.N.P., B.C.

INTRODUCTION

Lymphedema is a significant cause of decreased function and quality of life for many patients with breast cancer. It is estimated to occur in 25% of women with breast cancer with a range of 6% to 68%, depending on treatment (Yarbro, 2011). Because the risk for lymphedema persists for life, measures to prevent this complication should be considered in every patient's Survivor Care Plan as recommended by the Institute of Medicine (National Cancer Institute, 2015). This awareness and management of lymphedema is most effective early in cancer care and requires involvement on the part of both provider and patient. Surveillance for early occurrence of lymphedema and timely and effective intervention will reduce the risk for disability. Primary care providers and gynecologists are in a prime position to evaluate and direct care to improve outcomes for patients with breast cancer. The purpose of this article is to prepare providers and nurses for this task.

THE LYMPHATIC SYSTEM RELATIVE TO BREAST CANCER

The lymphatic system is a network of lymph vessels, lymph nodes, and lymphoid tissue distributed throughout the human body. The lymphatic system has three main functions: balancing fluid within the tissues, transporting cells involved in the immune response, and removing proteins and particles of cellular debris from the tissue spaces (Saito, 2013).

Lymph flow occurs in a relatively low pressure system. It begins by uptake of fluid from the interstitial space into tiny vessels. Pulsation of arteries and contraction of skeletal muscles help propel the fluid until it reaches larger lymph vessels. In these larger lymph vessels, smooth muscle actions move the lymph to superficial and deep lymph nodes, then into the venous system. The corresponding thoracic duct is the entry point for the chest wall, breast, and arm lymphatics into the venous circulation. Both superficial and deep lymph systems in the upper extremities merge in the axilla.

157

Lymphedema occurs when any disruption of this system causes lymphatic load to exceed transport capacity, pushing protein-rich fluid into the interstitial spaces (Mohler, 2015). In addition, because the lymphatic system transports leukocytes, antigens, and dendritic cells in mounting an immune response, disruption will decrease the body's ability to fight infection in the region normally fed by that portion of the lymphatic network (Saito, 2013).

In patients with breast cancer, both the disease and its treatment may increase the risk for lymphedema. Although most concern is directed at lymphedema in the arm because of the potential for loss of function, it also can occur in the chest wall in patients who have undergone mastectomy and, in some cases, in the remaining breast tissue after lumpectomy. Breast tumors can compress channels and nodes; tumor cells can infiltrate the channels. In addition, inflammation from infection or limb injury can adversely affect the lymphatic system's function.

Lymphedema also presents the risk for recurrent infection (National Cancer Institute, 2015). Surgical removal of lymph nodes and radiation therapy of an area of the lymphatics can damage the system, interrupting the flow of lymph (Mohler, 2015). This will be discussed in more detail below.

BREAST CANCER SURGERY AND LYMPHEDEMA RISK

Surgery for breast cancer is far less radical than it has been in the past, with today's treatment choices based on evidence and outcomes studies. The current focus is on minimizing deformity and long-range complications whenever possible, while achieving at least equivalent disease control.

An important example is the change in practice that ensued based on the results of the randomized, phase III clinical trial, the American College of Surgeons Oncology Group Z0011 (ACOSOG-Z0011) study. The ACOSOG-Z0011 study involved women with early stage (T1 to T2) breast cancer. All patients underwent lumpectomy (partial mastectomy) and breast irradiation. (Some patients also had systemic therapy at the discretion of their treating physicians.) Patients who were found to have metastatic cells in one or two sentinel lymph nodes (SLNs) on SLN dissection were randomized either to also undergo complete axillary lymph node dissection (ALND), or to receive no further axillary treatment. The study showed no significant decrease in survival with SNL dissection alone compared to complete ALND (Giuliano, 2011). This is encouraging news for many women.

In UpToDate 2015, Mohler and Mondry summarize that SLND carries a 64% lower risk for lymphedema than does ALND (Mohler, 2015).

The procedure for SLN biopsy usually involves using a nuclear medicine dye injected into the breast prior to surgery to identify the first "sentinel" nodes to which cancer would travel via lymph fluid. During surgery, a gamma probe is used to identify significant levels of activity in one to four nodes, and these are removed. If this method does not provide sufficient information, a blue dye can be injected in the operating room that will color the nodes. If neither provides adequate information, the surgeon is forced to perform axillary node dissection (Yarboro, 2011). The National Cancer Institute review notes that the degree of tissue disruption using SLND causes between a 5% and 17% risk of lymphedema (National Cancer Institute, 2015).

Axillary lymph node dissection usually involves removal of the level I-II nodes (below and underneath the pectoralis minor muscle), but may go on to level III (above the pectoralis minor muscle) if the surgeon has identified palpable or radiologic concern for disease presence in these areas. The number of nodes identified on pathologic examination of tissue removed by ALND usually is between 20 and 30 nodes. The National Cancer Institute reviews indicate that the risk for lymphedema after ALND ranges from 20% to 53% (National Cancer Institute, 2015).

Preoperative tumor location, extent of breast surgery, and postsurgical delayed healing, infection, seroma, and scarring may further damage the lymphatic tissue and increase an individual patient's risk for lymphedema. (Mohler, 2015).

OTHER CONTRIBUTING RISK FACTORS

Radiation

Axillary lymph nodes are often irradiated as part of regional treatment to prevent breast cancer recurrence. Tumor boards continue to debate complete ALND versus radiation of the ALNs or both for individuals with node-positive disease. The European Organisation for Research and Treatment of Cancer's 10981-22023 AMAROS trial showed similar risk reduction of recurrence as ALND in a select group, but with less lymphedema (Donker, 2014). In this study, half of the patients were randomly assigned—prior to SNL biopsy—to receive either ALND or axillary radiotherapy. Patients with a positive sentinel node received their previously assigned treatment and were followed for a median of ten years. The primary endpoint was five-year axillary recurrence; lymphedema was among the secondary endpoints.

At one year of follow up, 28% of patients (114 of 410) in the ALND group had clinical signs of lymphedema and 8% (32 of 410) had an increase of 10% or greater in the ipsilateral arm; in contrast, lymphedema was seen in 15% (62/410) of patients in the axillary radiotherapy group, and 6% (24/410) greater than 10% arm circumference increase. At year five, the lymphedema rates were 23% (76/328) in the ALND group and 11% (31/286) in the radiotherapy group. Arm circumference increases of greater than 10% at year five were 13% (42/328) in the ALND group and 5% (16/286) in the radiotherapy group (Donker, 2014).

There were no significant differences between treatment groups in disease-free survival and survival rates.

Although lymphedema often is considered a problem primarily in the arms of patients with breast cancer, it can also be seen in the breasts of patients who undergo partial mastectomy followed by radiation therapy (breast conserving therapy) and in the chest walls of patients who undergo mastectomy followed by chest wall radiation.

Obesity

It is known that the lymphatic system is involved in fat absorption and deposition, but the involvement of fat in lymphedema pathophysiology is just beginning to be understood. It has been observed that with weight gain, an arm with lymphedema accumulates fat more quickly than does tissue in the rest of the body, but loses fat more slowly when an individual experiences weight loss (Saito, 2013). Obesity is considered an independent risk factor for lymphedema (Mohler, 2015).

Infection

Lymph fluid in a patient with lymphedema is rich in protein and, thus, provides a medium for bacterial growth. As the lymphatic response is disabled, local bacterial and fungal infections can progress unchecked. In turn, the infection can further damage the lymphatics, causing a cycle that may become irreversible (Saito, 2013).

MONITORING FOR POSTSURGICAL SIGNS AND SYMPTOMS

Lymphedema typically progresses slowly, through a series of stages. Early diagnosis and intervention are important to prevent progression of the condition and worsening of signs and symptoms. The diagnosis of lymphedema in a patient who has undergone surgery for breast cancer usually can be made clinically, based on patient-reported symptoms and/or on an increased arm circumference measurement, although such changes may be quite subtle in the early stages of lymphedema. For example, a patient who has undergone ALND and presents with the complaint that her arm "feels heavy" may be experiencing tissue changes of stage 0 or may have early stage I lymphedema. Women also describe early symptoms as changes in sensation and range of motion (Armer, 2003).

Patients also should be asked if any activities bring on any of the signs or symptoms listed above for possible modification. It is not uncommon for patients to note some swelling after gardening, carrying groceries, or doing housework that resolves soon thereafter. Progressive planned exercise can help prevent this from occurring. Sudden dramatic onset of significant lymphedema has been observed clinically in patients who go from low activity to boat rowing for a weekend or who return to their prior weight lifting at the gym. This is because the sudden strain causes inflammation and injury to the tissue that can cause lymphedema (PDQ, 2015). However sudden onset, dramatic lymphedema should prompt an ultrasound to rule out deep vein thrombosis or a mass impeding flow.

DIAGNOSTIC MODALITIES

Clinical measurements should be used to document and support a diagnosis of lymphedema and guide management.

Tape measurement of arm circumference is a reasonable method of diagnosing lymphedema. Ideally, baseline measurements of specific anatomic landmarks should be obtained before surgery; the dominant limb often is somewhat larger at baseline due to differences in muscle mass development over time. Postsurgery, a difference of 2 cm between arms (corrected for presurgery differences) is considered significant (Mohler, 2015). Arm volume can be assessed by water displacement or optoelectronic volumetry, if equipment for such testing is readily available. A disadvantage of either arm circumference or volume measure is that lymphedema often has progressed to at least stage 1 before changes over baseline can be appreciated (Soran, 2014).

Lymphoscintigraphy is an imaging technique that requires tracers to monitor lymph flow at rest and after activity such as squeezing a ball for 20 minutes. Protocols vary among treatment centers. Lymphoscintigraphy can be useful in a patient who develops lymphedema after SLND for breast cancer; this imaging technique can identify the source and specific site of lymph flow obstruction.

Bioimpedance spectroscopy (BIS) measures extracellular fluid and has been used for many years in fitness evaluations of body composition. More recently, it has been validated as a reliable and accurate method to detect early changes of lymphedema (Warren, 2007). This device measures resistance to a small, painless, electrical current, passed through the limb: the higher the water content in the interstitial fluid, the lower the resistance. By comparing resistance in a patient's arm, lymphedema may be detected earlier than is possible using tape measurements of arm circumference.

In one prospective, single-center study comparing BIS and tape measure, 186 patients who had undergone ALND were divided into two groups: one group was followed with BIS and the other was monitored with tape measurements. In the first group, subclinical lymphedema (stage 0) was detected in 33% of patients who received early intervention; only 4.4% progressed to clinical lymphedema. In contrast, in the standard tape measurement group, none of the patients were identified at stage 0; clinical lymphedema (stage 1) was identified in 36.4% of patients. Thus, BIS allowed early detection and treatment that reduced clinical lymphedema from 36.4% to 4.4% (Soran, 2014).

A phase III, randomized trial currently is underway comparing BIS and arm circumference tape measurements (ClinicalTrials.gov). In this study, patients who have undergone breast cancer surgery are monitored with either BIS or tape measurements and receive intervention—use of a compression sleeve with gauntlet—as soon as the earliest signs of lymphedema occur. The primary end point is a reduction in the rate of progression with complex decongestive physiotherapy (CDP) with BIS versus standard tape measurements.

Meanwhile, experience in an ongoing clinical setting will be helpful in determining the optimum application of BIS. One BIS device that is small and easy to operate is being used at Comprehensive Breast Care at Pluta, part of the Wilmot Cancer Institute at the University of Rochester, New York. According to the protocol established for BIS at this center, a reading is done preoperatively to establish a baseline measurement; measurements are repeated at regular postoperative intervals, and additional readings are done if patients have new complaints or observations. Changes that are deemed significant, according to the manufacturer's guidelines, initiate a patient's referral to the occupational therapy department for additional evaluation and treatment. This tool also is used to monitor response to treatment. (No formal analysis of the experience with BIS at this center is available at this time, but observation of individual clinical cases has supported the benefit of using the BIS device.)

All patients who are monitored with this BIS device receive several reinforcements of education regarding lymphedema risk, prevention, and early detection. Increases in BIS measurements also prompt updated discussions about compliance with treatments, which will be will be further discussed in the following sections.

LYMPHEDEMA OF THE ARM: STAGES AND INTERVENTIONS

Lymphedema is considered primary if it is not directly caused by another medical condition. Secondary lymphedema is the result of a disruption to the lymphatic system due to surgical excision, radiation, or trauma. Impairment of the lymphatic system poses a risk for secondary lymphedema, which progresses in stages without prompt and effective intervention.

Impaired lymphatic flow poses an increased risk for bacterial or fungal infections in patients with any degree of lymphedema (Deng, 2014). Patients should be made aware of and monitored for signs and symptoms of infection. Mild skin redness without fever or pain is most likely not a sign of infection, but the patient should be observed while the lymphedema treatment regimen is re-evaluated. Prompt treatment of infection with appropriate antibiotics or antifungals is needed for acute episodes of cellulitis, lymphangitis, or erysipelas.

STAGE 0 (SUBCLINICAL) LYMPHEDEMA

Stage 0—also sometimes referred to as "pending lymphedema"—is clinically undetectable, with no visible changes to the arm, hand, or upper body. Patients may experience mild tingling or heaviness in the arm. Stage 0 lymphedema may persist for a long time—even up to years, before clinical symptoms develop. Stage 0 may be identified with the use of BIS (as discussed above).

STAGE 1 LYMPHEDEMA

At stage 1, lymphedema is highly reversible; spontaneous resolution can occur several times and over periods of years before symptoms persist without remission. Symptoms include the recent onset of mild swelling ("puffiness") and pitting in the soft tissue of the arm (Lawenda, 2009). Because lymphedema is pressure-dependent, pooling tends to occur in the areas of soft tissue, not at the joints. Another sign of early lymphedema is an out-of-normal bioelectrical impedance analysis result (Fu, 2013). This test directly measures fluid changes.

Stage 1 Intervention

- Stop the activity that triggered the edema.

- Elevate the involved arm much of the day and at night.

- Complete self-lymphatic stimulation. Self-lymphatic stimulation is a technique taught to patients to be completed at home, beyond clinic treatment. The patient begins with deep abdominal breathing, and progressively follows the lymphatic channels to the lymph nodes with a gentle hand-on technique.

If these measures result in resolution of lymphedema, reinforce that the compression sleeve is to be worn during the triggering activity. If the symptoms are not resolved, institute reduction measures as described for stage 2 lymphedema.

Impact of Stage 1 Lymphedema on Function/Quality of Life

Anecdotal reports indicate that functional limitations from stage 1 lymphedema are temporary and are related to treatment restrictions. In one report, a limb size change of 10% or less relative to preoperative baseline measurements did not affect the use of the involved arm in performing activities of daily living (O'Toole, 2015).

STAGE 2 LYMPHEDEMA

Stage 2 lymphedema is considered to be partially reversible, with signs and symptoms regressing to the level of stage 1 lymphedema; complete and long-term resolution is rare. The goal is reduction of stage 2 signs and symptoms followed by maintenance of stage 1 symptoms. Signs of stage 2 lymphedema include a measurable increase in the size of the arm, mild skin changes, a heavy feeling, skin sensation of tightness, and snug-feeling clothes and jewelry. The fluid is nonpitting and the tissue feels more spongy than in stage 1 (Lawenda, 2009). Symptoms of stage 2 lymphedema may persist for months to years, with noticeable and progressive arm size differences. The skin can become red and thickened over time due to decreased skin nutrition. The impairment to the immune function of the lymphatic system can lead to dermatologic infections, including cellulitis.

Stage 2 Intervention

Complete decongestive therapy (CDT) is the standard of care for stage 2 lymphedema intervention. This program includes impeccable skin hygiene; guided movement; therapist-administered, full-body, decongestive hands-on techniques; and serial compression with short stretch bandages. The patient is educated about the role of the lymphatic system in stage 2 lymphedema, and is taught how to perform more advanced self-lymphatic stimulation, to be performed for 20 minutes, twice a day.

The reduction technique of serial wrapping with short stretch bandages is demonstrated by the therapist. During the induction phase of reduction, the patient attends about four therapy visits over 2 weeks for initial therapist wrapping; the patient and/or her caregiver are taught the technique at these visits. During this phase, the bandages are worn at all times between therapy visits. Once the patient or caregiver can perform serial wrapping competently, the bandages should be unwrapped each evening and washed and allowed to dry overnight; the patient should sleep with the extremity elevated, and the bandages should be reapplied in the morning.

The lymphatic stimulation and self-drainage techniques are continued throughout the reduction program. Measurements are taken periodically, and adjustments to wrapping and the drainage techniques are made as indicated. Each application is with a specific graded tension that will ideally compress and reduce volume; the wraps are removed and reapplied at this reduced volume, creating a progressive reduction. Because of the increased demand that the reduction technique places on the lymphatic system, the patient should not participate in high-energy exercises and activities during the program.

Most patients can tolerate wearing bandages and a decrease in arm function for 1 month. Once reduction is achieved, the patient is referred to a medical supply store to be measured for custom garments, usually a full arm sleeve and glove with three-quarter digits. The patient continues to wrap until the garments arrive, typically 2 to 3 weeks later. Once the transition is made to the custom garments, the goal is containment of the current size of the arm. The garments should be worn every day, all day, as tolerated, for 3 months. At the 3-month follow-up visit, if there is good containment, as defined by no appreciable increase in size, periods out of the garment are slowly added into the daily routine.

Patient participation factors can negatively influence the success of the treatment. Currently, short stretch bandages and supplies can cost $100, and custom compression sleeves typically cost $250 with a glove costing $250 as well. Currently, these costs are not usually an insurance-covered expense. We have found that a significant number of patients are unable to participate in a lymphedema management program due to financial limitations. The time demand of daily donning, discomfort and limited movement related to wearing the wraps or garments, and social awkwardness all impact on successful symptom management. Occupational and physical therapists can become certified lymphedema therapists by attending and meeting standards in a multi-week, in-depth course. This advanced certification can be a referral guide; however, many very qualified therapists do not choose to become certified. A therapist who has a caseload dedicated to patients with lymphedema is likely to be a sound referral.

Impact of Stage 2 Lymphedema on Function/Quality of Life

Progression to stage 2 lymphedema is a life-altering event as it is considered to be not fully reversible. Daily routines are affected, lymphedema containment garments are visible to the patient and to others and may adversely affect self-perception. Activities must be monitored, and adherence to the risk reduction guidelines must become more rigid.

STAGE 3 LYMPHEDEMA

Stage 3 lymphedema is considered partially reversible with ongoing, significant intervention. In this stage, signs of stage 2 persist, and the edema is nonpitting with pooled areas forming lobules. There is an increase in the severity of the fibrotic response and other skin changes (Lawenda, 2009).The long-term stagnation of lymphatic movement in these areas provides a favorable environment for bacterial growth, and because the weight of the enlarged arm compromises movement, pumping of the lymphatic fluid is reduced. All of these factors combine to create a higher risk for serious dermatologic infections, including cellulitis.

Stage 3 Intervention

Reduction technique should be completed as described for stage 2 lymphedema. Full reduction to a plateau may take several months. At this point, if containment is not held with daytime garments, a pneumatic compression pump, a higher grade of pressure for daytime garments, and the use of nighttime garments are considered. Patients are counseled to monitor and restrict any activities that increase lymphedema symptoms. Fibrosis and firmness often are present; treatment for this symptom is described in the section on breast lymphedema, below.

Impact of Stage 3 Lymphedema on Function/Quality of Life

Following the recommendations to maintain containment at the current symptom level can limit work and home roles, such as child care activities and interactions. Women who can no longer participate in certain leisure activities with their families and friends, such as spending extended periods of time outdoors, exposed to heat and the sun, are deprived of such enjoyment.

A disproportionally large arm creates a clothing fit challenge. Often, women squeeze the affected arm into a sleeve to avoid wearing a completely oversized shirt (which is not recommended, as the pressure in clothing fabrics is inconsistent); some patients are forced to have their clothes tailored to accommodate the involved arm.

Jobs that require heavy, repetitive lifting in a warm and changeable environment such as warehouse, factory, or farming positions are challenging for patients with stage 3 lymphedema. Jobs that demand a high level of a rapid emergency response—such as driving a bus or working in certain health care environments—are discouraged.

However, each situation is individual, and whenever possible, efforts should be made to keep patients employed and active, perhaps with modifications.

BREAST LYMPHEDEMA

Breast lymphedema often presents after partial mastectomy and breast irradiation. Pooling, and therefore thickening, of lymphatic fluid tends to occur in the medial inferior aspect of the breast. The patient should be educated about the role of the lymphatic system relative to the breast. Encapsulation and compressive bras are recommended to lift and support the shape of the breasts, with an overlayer of compression. A chip bag with small pieces of multiple density foam is added to the bra over areas where firmness persists. Therapeutic ultrasound also may be considered to treat firm areas of the breast. These techniques also can be used on arm firmness secondary to lymphedema. Lymphedema itself is not painful. However the symptoms can be quite uncomfortable. Many women are self-conscious of the difference in breast size.

COMPREHENSIVE BREAST CARE AT PLUTA, WILMOT CANCER INSTITUTE, UNIVERSITY OF ROCHESTER MEDICAL CENTER

At the Compressive Breast Care at Pluta Cancer Center, we strive to educate women on the risk for postoperative lymphedema, both in the initial surgical oncology visit and the initial occupational therapy visit. This prepares the patient to begin therapeutic strategies immediately after surgery and take comfort in knowing what to expect.

At this visit, we focus on the first postoperative month. Our protocol includes guiding the patient in understanding the role of the lymphatic system and the possible impact of the surgical procedure. We discuss with patients the characteristics of postoperative edema versus lymphedema, and inform them that our guidelines are designed to minimize the risk for both.

Patients who are scheduled to have an axillary lymph node dissection return to occupational therapy approximately one month after their surgery postoperative date. The amount of education given on the possible progression of lymphedema, treatment options, and possible lifestyle impact is carefully considered to avoid overwhelming the patient with information about a complication that may not occur. Advanced education is given to women who indicate that they would find more detailed information reassuring.

The specific risk reduction strategies we—and many other centers—use are not validated by randomized, controlled scientific studies, but are based on widely used, long-standing practices that are reinforced by expert guidance from the American Cancer Society (American Cancer Society, 2015) and The Lymphedema Network (The Lymphedema Network, 2015).

At our center, recommendations for the first month following surgery are to engage in light activities only until the drains are removed or for approximately 2 weeks. For the remainder of the first month, activities can be performed as tolerated. The arm on the affected side should be propped comfortably on progressively higher surfaces (such as stacked pillows), as tolerated. The goal is to raise the arm until the hand is well above the level of the heart; once this position is achieved, the patient should open and close the hand intermittently. Movement about the household is encouraged. Needle sticks, blood pressure monitoring, and any trauma to the involved arm should be avoided. Baseline circumferential measurements are taken.

Following axillary lymph node dissection, patients are counseled to consider advanced risk reduction practices including those listed below. However, it is important to remember that these are recommendations for risk reduction only and should be balanced against quality of life.

- Wear an arm compression sleeve during high-altitude air travel and during or directly after high exertion activities or activities that are beyond a patient's known, normally tolerated routine.

- No specific exercises or activities are prohibited. Exercise does not increase the risk when a regimen progresses gradually and without symptoms, indicating that lymphedema is contained. In fact, numerous studies have shown that participation in a well-established exercise regime can decrease the risk for lymphedema.

- Compression garment wear during extended, multiple-hour car rides is recommended. Getting out of the car periodically for full body movement is also advised.

- Extremes in heat are to be minimized. For example, patients should spend no more than 15 minutes in a hot tub.

- Repetitive skin damage should be minimized, including dryness, scratches, minor cuts, and burns. This includes absolute avoidance of intravenous (IV) placement, blood draws, and injections in the affected arm. (If lymph nodes have been removed in both arms, clinical judgment should determine whether to access veins in the lower extremities, or use the arm with the least nodes removed. For repeated venous access, such as for chemotherapy, an implanted port may be preferred.)

- Constrictive clothing, jewelry, purse and bra straps, and blood pressure cuffs should be avoided. Clinically, sometimes a choice needs to be made about where to obtain an accurate blood pressure in women who have had nodal surgery on both arms. If a woman has had an axillary dissection on the left and only one-to-two nodes removed on the right, a quick manual blood pressure taken on the right without pumping as high or remaining as high as automatic cuffs would result in a lower risk of injury.

SUMMARY

Whatever our specific role, health care providers will encounter breast cancer survivors. Lymphedema of the arm or breast may occur at any point of diagnosis, treatment, or survivorship. Patients require education regarding prevention, careful observation, and early reporting of signs and symptoms of lymphedema. Patient knowledge combined with providers' assessment of history and available measurements, along with clinical examination, increases patients' chances for earlier detection of lymphedema. Earlier detection and treatment, perhaps even at a subclinical level, will minimize a potentially life-altering complication for breast cancer survivors.

REFERENCES

1. American Cancer Society (2015). Retrieved from http://www.cancercare.org/tagged/lymphedema, on May 24, 2015. The Lymphedema Network (2015). Retrieved from http://www.lymphnet.org/healthyhabits, on May 24, 2015.

2. Armer, JM, Radina ME, Porock D, and Culbertson SD (2003). Predicting breast cancer-related lymphedema using self-reported symptoms. Nursing Research, 52 (6):370-379.

3. Complete Decongestive Therapy, October 1, 2012, retrieved from http://www.breastcancer.org/treatment/lymphedema/treatments/cdt on May 24, 2015.

4. Deng J, Fu MR, Armer JM, Cormier JN, Radina ME, Thiadens SR, Weiss J, Tuppo CM, Dietrich MS, and Ridner SH (2015). Factors associated with reported infection and lymphedemasymptoms among individuals with extremity lymphedema. Rehabilitation Nursing, 40(5):310-319.

5. Donker M, van Tienhoven G, Straver ME, Meijnen P, van de Velde CJ, Mansel RE Cataliotti L, Westenberg AH, Klinkenbiljl JH, Orzalesi L, Bouma WH, van der Mijle HC, Nieuwenhuijzen GA, Veltkamp SC, Slaets L, Duez NJ, de Graaf PW, van Dalen T, Marinelli A, Rijna H, Snoj M, Bundred JK, Merkus JW, Belkacemi Y,Petignat P, Schinagl DA, Coens C, Messina CG, Bogaerts J, Rutgers EJ (2014). Radiotherapy or surgery of the axilla after a positive sentinel node in breast cancer (EORTC 10981-22023 AMAROS): A randomised, multicenter, open-label, phase 3 non-inferiority trial. Lancet Oncology, 15(12):1303-1310.

6. Fu MR, Cleland CM, Guth AA, Kayal M, Haber J, Cartwright F, Kleinman R, Kang Y, Scagliola J, and Axelrod D (2013). L-dex ratio in detecting breast cancer related lymphedema: Reliability, sensitivity, and specificity. Lymphology, 46(2):85-96.

7. Giuliano AE, Hunt K, Ballman K, Beitsch P, Whitworth P, Blumencranz P, Leitch M, Saha S, McCall L, and Morrow M, MD (2011). Axillary Dissection vs No Axillary Dissection in Women with Invasive Breast Cancer and Sentinel Node Metastasis (ACOSOG Z11 Trial). Journal of the American Medical Association, 305(6):569-575.

8. Lawenda BD, Mondry TE, Johnstone PA (2009). Lymphedema: a primer on the identification and management of a chronic condition in oncologic treatment. CA: A Cancer Journal for Clinicians, 59(1):8-24.

9. Mohler E and Mondry TE (2015). Clinical manifestations and diagnosis of lymphedema. Up to Date, 2015.retrieved from http://www.uptodate.com/contents/clinical-manifestations-and-diagnosis-of- lymphedema on March 14, 2015.

10. National Cancer institute. At the National Institute of Health. Lymphedema (PDQ) Health Professional Version. Retrieved from http://www.cancer.gov/about- cancer/treatment/side-effects/lymphedema/lymphedema-hp-pdq on April 21, 2015.

11. NLN Medical Advisory Committee (2011). Position Statement of the National Lymphedema Network Updated February 2011. Topic: The Diagnosis and Treatment of Lymphedema. NLN. 116 New Montgomery Street Suite 235. San Francisco, CA 94105. www.lymphnet.org

12. O'Toole JA, Ferguson CM, Swaroop MN, Horick N, Skolny MN, Brunelle CL, Miller CL, Jammallo LS, Specht MC, and Taghian AG (2015). The impact of breast cancer-related lymphedema on the ability to perform upper extremity activities of daily living. Breast Cancer Research and Treatment, 150(2):381-388.

13. PDQ Supportive and Palliative Care Editorial Board. Lymphedema (PDQ®): Health Professional Version (2015). In: PDQ Cancer Information Summaries. Bethesda (MD): National Cancer Instititute (US); 2002-.Available from: https://www.ncbi.nlm.nih.gov/books/NBK65803/.

14. Saito Y, Nakagami H, Kaneda Y, and Ryuichi (2013). Lymphedema and Therapeutic Lymphangiogeniesis. Biomedical Research International, 2013: 804675. Published online 2013 Oct 9. Doi 10.1155/2013/804675 retrieved from http://www.ncbi.nlm.nih.gov/pmc/articles/PMC3810055/ on April 14, 2015.

15. Soran A, Ozmen T, McGuire KP, Diego E, McAuliffe P, Bonaventura M, Ahrendt G, DeGore L, and Johnson R (2014). The importance of detection of subclinical lymphedema for the prevention of breast cancer-related clinical lymphedema after axillary lymph node dissection: A prospective observational study. Lymphatic Research and Biology, 12(4):289-294.

16. Yarbro C, Wujcik D, and Gobel B (2010). Cancer Nursing Principles and Practice, (Ed. 7). Sudbury MA: Jones and Bartlett.

17. Warren AG, Janz BA, Slavin SA, Borud LJ (2007). The Use of Bioimpedance Analysis to Evaluate Lymphedema. Annals of Plastic Surgery, 58(5):541-543.

SLEEP DISORDERS IN
BREAST CANCER SURVIVORS

Jayne Knowlton, M.S., O.T.R. /L. and Manisha Sheth, O.T.D., O.T.R./L.

Introduction

Sleep problems, inadequate sleep duration, poor sleep quality, poor sleep timing, and sleep disorders are important public health problems that impact more than 70 million people in the United States (U.S.) and lead to an 11% to 20% increase in healthcare costs (Otte, 2016). Sleep problems also are one of the top five most burdensome lingering issues in breast cancer survivors (BCS). It is well documented that 67% to 90% of BCS report sleep problems. Sleep problems are long–term issues for BCS, commonly experienced for as many as ten years post treatment (Otte, 2016).

In this chapter, we will provide an overview of the impact and management of sleep disorders. Because sleep disorders are so prevalent among menopausal women as well as those living with the challenges of breast cancer, the recommendations provided here apply equally to both.

Insufficient or poor quality sleep is the most common complaint in those with cancer–related insomnia (CRI). Yet, sleep disorders are not unique to BCSs and, in fact, impact many women as they progress from their reproductive years into menopause.

Despite growing evidence that adequate sleep, like adequate nutrition and physical activity, is vital to our well-being, people are sleeping less. The nonstop "24/7" nature of the world today encourages longer or nighttime work hours and offers continual access to entertainment and other activities. To keep up, people cut back on sleep. A common myth is that people can learn to get by on little sleep (such as less than six hours a night) with no adverse effects. Research suggests that adults need at least seven to eight hours of sleep each night to be well rested. More than one-third of adults report daytime sleepiness so severe that it interferes with work, driving, and social functioning at least a few days each month. Evidence also shows that children and adolescents' sleep is shorter than recommended. These trends have been linked to increased exposure to electronic media (National Sleep Foundation, 2014).

Sleep insufficiency, defined as not obtaining restorative sleep, is a public health crisis in the U.S. with resulting negative economic consequences due to lower productivity, increased absenteeism, decreased job performance, increased healthcare utilization, and potential injury (American Sleep Association, 2016). It is believed to result in an annual cost of $16 billion in healthcare expenses and $50 billion in lost productivity (NIH, 2011).

Normal Physiology of Sleep

Sleep is defined as a recurring, reversible neurobehavioral state of relative perceptual disengagement from, and unresponsiveness to, the environment. Sleep in humans is typically accompanied by "postural recumbency, behavioral quiescence, [and] closed eyes" (Carskadon, 2005). Table 1 shows the recommended hours of sleep for age groups from birth to older adult. Note that adults 18 to 64 years should receive seven to nine hours of sleep each night.

Age	Recommended Hours of Sleep
Newborn (0 to 2 months)	12 to 18 hours
Infant (3 to 11 month)	14 to 15 hours
Toddler (1 to 3 years)	12 to 14 hours
Preschooler (3 to 5 years)	11 to 13 hours
School-age children (5 to 10 years)	10 to 11 hours
Teen (10 to 17 years)	8.5 to 9.25 hours
Adult (18 to 64 years)	7 to 9 hours
Older adult (65 +)	7 to 8 hours

Table 1. Recommended Hours of Sleep Throughout the Lifespan (American Sleep Association, 2016).

During a person's normal sleeping hours, he or she typically will progress through five sleep cycles of approximately 90 minutes, as illustrated in Figure 1. There are two fundamental sleep types that occur in each cycle, and a different area in the brain regulates each. When the person is engaged in active dreaming, this is called rapid eye movement (REM) sleep. In REM sleep, breathing becomes faster, irregular, and shallow, the eyes jerk quickly in various directions, and limb muscles become temporarily paralyzed. Heart rate increases, blood pressure rises, and males may develop penile erections. When people awaken during REM sleep, they often describe bizarre and illogical tales, namely dreams. Non-rapid eye movement (NREM) sleep is dreamless sleep. In contrast to REM sleep, the person's breathing and heart rate are slow and regular, blood pressure is low, and the sleeper mostly is still (American Sleep Association, 2016).

In each sleep cycle, the individual progresses through NREM stages 1 through 4, culminating in REM sleep, also depicted in Figure 1. Stage 1 is light sleep. The person drifts in and out of sleep and can be awakened easily. The eyes move very slowly, and muscle activity is diminished. People awakened from Stage 1 sleep often remember fragmented visual images. Many also experience sudden muscle contractions called **hypnic myoclonia**, often preceded by a sensation of starting to fall. These sudden movements are similar to the way a person jumps when startled. During Stage 2, eye movements cease, and brain waves, as measured by an electroencephalogram, become slower with occasional bursts of rapid waves called **sleep spindles.** Extremely slow brain waves called **delta waves that are** interspersed with smaller, faster waves begin to appear in Stage 3. The brain produces delta waves almost exclusively in Stage 4. It is very difficult to wake someone during Stages 3 and 4, which together are called **deep sleep, also called slow-wave sleep.** There is no eye movement or muscle activity. People awakened during deep sleep do not adjust immediately and often feel groggy and disoriented for several minutes after they wake up. Some children experience bedwetting, night terrors, or sleepwalking during deep sleep. A person spends almost 50 percent of total sleep time in Stage 2 NREM, about 20 percent in REM, and the remaining 30 percent in Stages 1, 3, and 4 NREM (American Sleep Association, 2016).

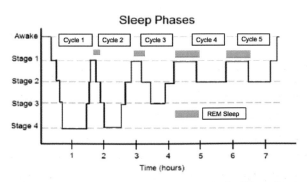

Figure 1. Sleep Cycle. Stages of sleep in the sleep cycle (Wikimedia Commons, 2013).

Table 2. Functions of Sleep

1.	Conservation of energy
2.	Restoration of tissues and growth. During the first hour of sleep, growth hormone excretion, cell mitosis, and protein syntheses are increased.
3.	Thermoregulation
4.	Regulation of emotions. In humans, sleep deprivation causes disturbances of emotional behavior such as concentration, interest of distinct goals.
5.	Neural maturation. The percentage of REM sleep of total sleep time decreases with age.
6.	Memory and learning. There is information transfer between the cortex and hippocampus during sleep that realizes the fixation of memory traces, or during REM sleep, the insignificant bindings are abolished.

Abbas A (2008). Rest and Sleep. Retrieved from Fundamentals of Nursing Department, College of Nursing, University of Baghdad: www.conursing. uobaghdad.edu.iq/uploads/others/.../ali/rest%20and%20sleep.pdf

Factors Affecting Sleep (Sinha, 2009)

The quality and quantity of sleep are affected by a number of factors. The quality of sleep refers to the individual's ability to stay asleep and to get an appropriate amount of REM and NREM sleep. Quantity of sleep is the total time the individual sleeps.

Developmental Considerations. Variations in sleep patterns are related to age. According to the 2004 National Sleep Foundation (NSF) Survey, children sleep less than the recommended time for their age group.

Motivation. A desire to be wakeful and alert helps overcome sleepiness. For example, a tired person may be wakeful and alert when attending an interesting play or concert. The opposite also is true. When there is minimal motivation to be awake, sleep generally follows.

Culture. An individual's cultural beliefs and practices can influence rest and sleep. Methods to enhance or foster sleep also may be culturally influenced. For example, an older Asian patient may choose herbal tea rather than a sleeping medication to promote or improve relaxation and sleep.

Lifestyles and Habits. Various lifestyle factors can affect a person's ability to sleep well. People working a shift other than the day shift must recognize their priorities or sleep difficulties may occur. Based on circadian cycle, the body prepares for sleep at night by decreasing the body temperature and releasing melatonin.

Physical Activity and Exercise. Activity and exercise increase fatigue and, in many instances, promote relaxation that is followed by sleep. It appears that physical activity increases both REM and NREM sleep. Moderate exercise is a healthy way to promote sleep, but exercise that occurs within a two-hour interval before normal bedtime can hinder sleep and decrease the quality of sleep.

Dietary Habits. It has long been believed that the dietary amino acid L-tryptophan acts to promote sleep. A small, protein-containing snack before bedtime used to be recommended for patients with insomnia. Protein may actually increase alertness and concentration, whereas carbohydrates appear to affect brain serotonin levels and promote calmness and relaxation.

Alcohol Intake. Alcoholic beverages, when used in moderation, appear to induce sleep in some people. However, large quantities have been found to limit REM and delta sleep. This effect may partially explain the phenomena of hangover after excessive alcohol consumption.

Caffeine-Containing Beverages. Caffeine is a central nervous system stimulant. For many people, beverages containing caffeine interfere with the ability to fall asleep, e.g., coffee, tea, most cola drinks, and chocolates.

Smoking. Nicotine has a stimulating effect on the body, and smokers often have more difficulty falling asleep than non-smokers do. Smokers usually are easily aroused and often describe themselves as light sleepers. By refraining from smoking after the evening meal, the person usually sleeps better; moreover, many former smokers report that their sleeping patterns improved once they stopped smoking.

Environmental Factors. Environment can promote or hinder sleep. Most people sleep best in their usual home environment. Sleeping in a strange or new environment tends to influence both REM and NREM. Stage 1 is the lightest and stages 3 and 4 are the deepest. As a result, louder noises are needed to awake a person in stages 3 and 4.

Psychological Stress. Illness and various life situations can cause psychological stress, which may disturb sleep. Psychological stress affects sleep in two ways.

- The person experiencing stress may find it difficult to obtain the amount of sleep he or she needs.

- Rapid eye movement sleep decreases in amount, which tends to increase anxiety and stress.

Effects of Sleep Deprivation

Sleep deprivation has serious health impacts, both in the short and long term. The main effect of sleep deprivation is excessive daytime sleepiness, which can lead to traffic accidents and workplace injuries (Sutter Health Palo Alto Medical Foundation, 2015). Table 3 lists the serious impacts of sleep deprivation.

Table 3. The Ways That Sleep Deprivation Can Impact a Person's Health (Sutter Health Palo Alto Medical Foundation, 2015).

Short-Term Impact	Long-Term Impact
• Anxiety	• High blood pressure
• Drowsiness, leading to drowsy driving	• Heart attack
• Forgetfulness	• Stroke
• Distractibility	• Obesity
• Decreased performance and alertness	• Type 2 diabetes
• Memory and cognitive impairment	• Depression and mood disorder
• Stressed relationship	• Poor quality of life
• Occupational injury	
• Automobile injury	

SLEEP ASSESSMENT (ABBAS 2008)

Primary care physicians can perform sleep assessment as a part of the diagnosis process when a client first reports sleep problems. Sleep assessment also can serve as an essential part of the management process of sleep deprivation. Discussion of sleep habits can be included as a part of the regular health history. Any client acknowledging a sleep disturbance should be thoroughly assessed to determine his/her:

- sleep routine,
- sleep alteration,
- types of sleep disturbances, and impact of sleep problems on his/her daily routine.

Questions regarding the patient's usual sleep pattern should include:

- nature of sleep (restful, uninterrupted),
- quality of sleep (usual sleep pattern, schedule, hours of sleep, and feeling on waking),
- sleep environment (description of room, number of people sleeping in one room, temperature, noise level and light in the room),
- associated factors (bedtime routine, use of sleep medication or any other sleep inducer), and
- opinion of sleep (adequate, inadequate, or problematic).

Questions regarding altered sleep patterns are intended to discover information such as:

- the nature of the problem (inability to fall asleep, difficulty remaining asleep, inability to fall asleep after awakening).
- the quality of the problem (number of hours of sleep versus number of hours spent trying to sleep, total number of hours of sleep a night, duration and frequency of daytime nap, and number of wakings per sleep period at night).
- environmental factors such as the bed, level of noise, lighting in the bedroom, surrounding stimulation, and sleeping partner's sleep habits.
- associated factors such as time and type (heavy or light) of the last meal before bed, activity prior to bed, level of stress, anxiety and pain, recent illness or surgery.

- the effect of problems such as fatigue, irritability and confusion on sleep (E Provide, Dysfunctional Beliefs And Attitudes About Sleep - *16 (DBAS-16)2007e*).

Some commonly used standardized sleep assessment tools are:

- The Epworth Sleeping Scale (Murray, n.d.),
- The Pittsburgh Sleep Quality Index (PSQI),
- The dysfunctional beliefs and attitudes about sleep brief version (DBAS-16) (Morin, 2007),
- (E Provide, Dysfunctional Beliefs And Attitudes About Sleep - *16 (DBAS-16)* (2007e),
- The Insomnia Severity Index (Morin,2011), and
- Glasgow Sleep Effort Scale (Broomfield and Espie, 2005).

Additional links for physicians:

http://sleepdisorders.sleepfoundation.org/chapter-1-normal-sleep/sleep-assessment-evaluation-primary-care-tools/

COMMON SLEEP DISORDERS (O'SHEA, 2015)

Insomnia

Causes: High levels of stress, certain medications, anxiety or depression. Drugs or alcohol abuse.

Symptoms: Difficulty falling asleep and then maintaining that sleep. While everyone has a bad night of sleep now and then, insomnia is a chronic issue, not acute.

Treatment: Cognitive behavioral therapy and/or medication often are prescribed.

Occurrence: About one-third of all Americans suffer from insomnia.

Sleep Apnea

Causes: A complete or partial blockage of the throat.

Symptoms: Daytime sleepiness, morning headaches, and—as any person who has attempted to sleep beside someone with sleep apnea can attest—excessively loud snoring. Apnea may cause you to stop breathing multiple times per night.

Treatment: The most common treatment for sleep apnea is a CPAP (continuous positive airway pressure) machine, which keeps a person's throat open via a steady stream of air.

Occurrence: About one in five adults suffers from at least a mild form of sleep apnea.

Restless Leg Syndrome (RLS)

Causes: In most cases, doctors do not know the cause of RLS; however, they suspect that genes play a role. Nearly half of all people with RLS also have a family member with the condition.

Other factors associated with the development or worsening of RLS include:

- Chronic diseases: Certain chronic diseases and medical conditions, including iron deficiency, Parkinson's disease, kidney failure, diabetes, and peripheral neuropathy, often include symptoms of RLS. Treating these conditions may give some relief from RLS symptoms,

- Medications: Some types of medications, including anti-nausea drugs, antipsychotic drugs, some antidepressants, and cold and allergy medications containing sedating antihistamines, may worsen symptoms, and

- Pregnancy: Some women experience RLS during pregnancy, especially in the last trimester. Symptoms usually go away within a month after delivery.

Other factors, including alcohol use and sleep deprivation, may trigger symptoms or make them worse. Improving sleep or eliminating alcohol use in these cases may relieve symptoms.

Symptoms: An irresistible urge to move the limbs, not just the legs. It often occurs in the evening or during periods of rest.

Treatment: Regular exercise, reduction in caffeine and alcohol. For severe cases, medication can be prescribed.

Occurrence: About 10% of the population suffers from RLS. It's more common in women.

REM Sleep Behavior Disorder

Causes: The mechanism in the brain that prevents motor movement while sleeping doesn't function properly.

Symptoms: Sudden and intense movement during sleep. People with REM sleep behavior disorder have been known to thrash in bed and even jump out of bed.

Treatment: Medication often is advised.

Occurrence: Extremely rare; less than one percent of the population.

Narcolepsy

Causes: Abnormalities in the parts of the brain that control REM sleep.

Symptoms: While people with narcolepsy can suddenly fall asleep at the most inopportune moments, most spend their days in a disassociated middle ground of sleep.

Treatment: Medication often is advised.

Occurrence: Less than 200,000 adults are diagnosed per year.

Sleepwalking

Causes: Lack of sleep or inefficient sleep. Some medications. Illness or fever.

Symptoms: Walking while sleeping.

Treatment: Reducing liquids near bedtime. A quiet sleep environment and maintaining a regular sleep schedule.

Occurrences: A surprise aspect of sleepwalking is that it's most common in children, and no one is quite sure why. Nonetheless, nocturnal sleep-related eating disorder may occur during sleepwalking as a possible explanation for this phenomenon.

Sleep Terrors

Causes: Sleep deprivation, illness, and/or some medications.

Symptoms: Screaming and violent, short bursts of movement during sleep. When a person has a sleep terror episode they aren't fully awake; therefore, it can be extremely difficult to calm them down once they do wake up.

Treatment: Improve sleep environment, medication is given if the terrors are extreme.

Occurrences: Most commonly impacts children; few adults suffer from this disorder. Those with post-traumatic stress disorder (PTSD) are more likely to suffer from sleep terrors.

Bruxism (Teeth Grinding)

Causes: Most experts blame excessive stress and anxiety.

Symptoms: Headaches and/or a sore jaw when waking in the morning. Complaints from annoyed bedmates.

Treatment: Avoid chewing any items that aren't food, as it trains the jaw to clench. Most people with bruxism end up getting fitted with a mouth guard that can be provided by a dentist.

Occurrence: About 45 million Americans.

INTERVENTION FOR SLEEP DEPRIVATION

Pharmacologic Interventions for Sleep Deprivation

Listed below are some drugs that can be used to treat insomnia.

- Zolpidem (Ambien®, Intermezzo®)
- Eszopiclone (Lunesta®)
- Ramelteon (Rozerem®)
- Zaleplon (Sonata®)
- Doxepine (Silenor™)
- Benzodiazepines
- Antidepressants
- Over-the-counter sleep aids: Most of these sleeping pills are antihistamines and allergy medications.

Non-pharmacologic Interventions (Siebern, 2012)

Cognitive Behavioral Therapy for Insomnia

Cognitive Behavioral Therapy for Insomnia (CBTI) is a short-term treatment that includes four to eight sessions on average and adopts a multi-component approach, which typically includes sleep restriction, stimulus control, cognitive therapy, sleep hygiene, and relaxation training.

Sleep Diary: A log the patient keeps of how many hours are slept each night, how many awakenings during the night and their durations, the time taken to fall asleep, how well rested the patient felt upon awakening, and how sleepy the patient felt during the day. Factors affecting sleep such as the number of caffeinated or alcoholic drinks consumed and nap or exercise times and lengths also may be recorded (National Sleep Foundation, 2018).

Sample **Sleep Diary**

One of the best ways you can tell if you are getting enough good quality sleep, and whether you have signs of a sleep disorder, is by keeping a sleep diary. Use this sample diary to get started.
—Source: NHLBI

		Mon*	Tues	Wed	Thurs	Fri	Sat	Sun
Name								
	Today's date (include month/day/year):							
Complete in the Morning	Time I went to bed last night:	11 p.m.						
	Time I woke up this morning:	7 a.m.						
	No. of hours slept last night:	8						
	Number of awakenings and	5 times						
	total time awake last night:	2 hours						
	How long I took to fall asleep last night:	30 mins.						
	How awake did I feel when I got up this morning? 1—Wide awake 2—Awake but a little tired 3—Sleepy	2						
Complete in the Evening	Number of caffeinated drinks (coffee, tea, cola) and time when I had them today:	1 drink at 8 p.m.						
	Number of alcoholic drinks (beer, wine, liquor) and time when I had them today:	2 drinks 9 p.m.						
	Naptimes and lengths today:	3:30 p.m. 45 mins.						
	Exercise times and lengths today:	None						
	How sleepy did I feel during the day today? 1—So sleepy had to struggle to stay awake during much of the day 2—Somewhat tired 3—Fairly alert 4—Wide awake	1						
		* This column shows example diary entries—use as a model for your own diary notes						

Sleep Restriction Therapy: Sleep restriction therapy aims to limit the time spent in bed to no more than the actual time spent sleeping and to increase sleep efficiency by prolonging sleep time. Restricting the time spent in bed creates a mild sleep deprivation and can promote an earlier sleep onset, more effective and deeper sleep, and less night-by-night variability in the quality and quantity of sleep. This decreases insomnia and creates confidence in the ability to regain natural sleep (National Sleep Foundation, 2018).

A typical sleep restriction protocol includes
(National Sleep Foundation, 2018):

1.   Determine the individual's average total sleep time (ATST) per night (this can be calculated from a sleep diary that has been filled out for one week if relatively representative of the person's usual routine).

2.   Restrict the individual's time in bed each night to the ATST.

3.   Establish a fixed bedtime depending on the desired wake time in the morning, and do not permit any sleep to occur outside of the sleep window. (Do not, however, reduce time spent in bed to less than 4.5 hours per night, as this can lead to noncompliance with the sleep restriction therapy.)

4.   Monitor daily sleep efficiency, which is calculated by the total sleep time (TST) / time spent in bed multiplied by 100.

5.   5.Extend the time spent in bed by 15 minutes when the weekly average sleep efficiency exceeds 90 percent. Reduce the time spent in bed by 15 minutes when the weekly average sleep efficiency falls below 80 percent.

Stimulus Control

The main objective of stimulus control is to have the patient limit the amount of time spent awake in bed and re-associate the bed and bedroom with sleep in order to regulate sleep–wake schedules. The guidelines that are discussed with the patient include the following: 1) only going to bed when sleepy; 2) using the bed and bedroom only for sleep and sexual activity; 3) leaving the bed and bedroom if unable to fall asleep for longer than 15 to 20 minutes, returning only when sleepy; and 4) keeping a fixed wake time in the morning every day, which will help the patient acquire a consistent sleep and wake rhythm. These instructions are designed to help re-establish the bed and bedroom as strong cues for sleep.

Cognitive Therapy

Cognitive therapy is designed to challenge maladaptive beliefs and attitudes that serve to maintain insomnia. Worrying, faulty attributions, or unrealistic expectations of sleep may lead to increased emotional distress and, thus, lead to additional sleep disturbance, causing a vicious cycle. It is believed that challenging dysfunctional thoughts associated with sleep will decrease the anxiety and arousal associated with insomnia.

Sleep Hygiene

Sleep hygiene consists of recommending a variety of behaviors and tending to environmental factors (e.g., light, bedroom temperature) that are conducive to sleep. Examples of sleep hygiene instructions include avoiding heavy meals close to bedtime, limiting caffeine products throughout the day, avoiding alcohol to aid sleeping, avoiding smoking close to bedtime, avoiding naps during the daytime, and avoiding vigorous exercise close to bed time. Two approaches are recommended when delivering sleep hygiene instructions. One involves reviewing all sleep hygiene instructions with the patient using a didactic or Socratic approach. Another approach that is used more frequently involves assessing current sleep hygiene practices that the patient is implementing already, and tailoring intervention only to relevant behaviors that present as problems for the patient.

Relaxation Training

Learning relaxation techniques can be effective in reducing physiologic hyperarousal in the patient. Research suggests that relaxation is especially effective in helping with sleep initiation. Relaxation practice involves practicing relaxation techniques during the day, prior to bedtime, and also in the middle of the night, if the patient is unable to fall back asleep. Common relaxation techniques include progressive muscle relaxation, which involves alternately tensing and relaxing different muscle groups in the body; deep breathing techniques, which involve diaphragmatic breathing; body scanning, which involves focusing on a body-part sequence that covers the whole body; and autogenic training, which involves visualizing a peaceful scene and repeating autogenic phrases to deepen the relaxation response. Use of mindfulness-based therapy for insomnia, which is based on mindfulness mediation, guided imagery, and biofeedback, also can be incorporated into the treatment.

CONCLUSION

Despite the high prevalence of sleep disorders and their significant consequences, sleep complaints often are not addressed by primary care physicians. To date, the United States Preventive Services Task Force, the American Academy of Family Physicians, and the Centers for Disease Control and Prevention have not recommended routine screening for sleep disorders. In addition, limited time, lack of reimbursement, and high demand may be factors that hinder the provision of preventive health services by primary care physicians (Senthilvel, 2011).

Sleep, like nutrition and physical activity, is a critical determinant of health and well-being. Prevention and intervention strategies that address sleep needs at the level of the individual, family, and population lie within the scope of practice for any healthcare professionals (Green, 2015). This chapter on sleep hygiene will assist physicians to efficiently identify patients at risk for common sleep disorders and intervene effectively in primary care.

REFERENCES

1. Abbas A (2008). Rest and Sleep. Retrieved from Fundamentals of Nursing Department, College of Nursing, University of Baghdad: www.conursing.uobaghdad.edu.iq/uploads/others/.../ali/rest%20and%20sleep.pdf

2. American Sleep Association (2016). What is sleep? Retrieved from American Sleep Association: https://www.sleepassociation.org/patients-general-public/what-is-sleep/

3. AOTA (n.d.). Occupational Therapy's Role in Sleep. Retrieved August 4, 2016, from The American Occupational Therapy Association (AOTA): http://www.aota.org/about-occupational-therapy/professionals/hw/sleep.aspx

4. Broomfield N and Espie C (2005). Towards a valid, reliable measure of sleep effort. Journal of Sleep Research, 14(4):401-407.

5. Carskadon MA and Dement WC (2005). Normal human sleep: An overview (Chapter 2). In: MH Kryger, T Roth, and WC Dement, (Eds.). Principles and Practice of Sleep Medicine, (Ed. 4). Philadelphia: Elsevier, 13-23.

6. Dement W (2015, n.d.). Sleep: In Words. Retrieved August 4, 2016, from End-Your-Sleep-Deprivation: http://www.end-your-sleep-deprivation.com/quotes-about-sleep.htmlE Provide (2007e). Dysfunctional Beliefs And Attitudes About Sleep - *16 (DBAS-16)*. Retrieved from E Pprovide: https://eprovide.mapi-trust.org/instruments/dysfunctional-beliefs-and-attitudes-about-sleep-16

7. Green A, Brown C, and Iwama M (2015). An Occupational Therapist's Guide to Sleep and Sleep Problems. London: Jessica Kingsley Publishers.

8. HealthyPeople.gov (2016, September 12). Sleep health. Retrieved September 12, 2016, from HealthyPeople.gov: https://www.healthypeople.gov/2020/topics-objectives/topic/sleep-health

9. Induru R and Walsh D (2014). Cancer-related Insomnia. American Journal of Hospice and Palliative Medicine, 31(7):777-785.

10. Morin CM (2011). My health.va.gov. Retrieved from Insomnia Severity Index: www.myhealth.va.gov

11. Murray D (n.d.). The Epworth Sleepiness Scale. Retrieved from The Epworth Sleepiness Scale: http://epworthsleepinessscale.com/about-the-ess/

12. National Institute of Health (NIH) (2012, February 22). Why is Sleep Important. Retrieved from National Institute of Health (NIH): http://www.nhlbi.nih.gov/health/health-topics/topics/sdd/why

13. National Institute of Health (2011, August). Your guide to healthy sleep. Retrieved from National Institute of Health: https://www.nhlbi.nih.gov/files/docs/public/sleep/healthy_sleep.pdf

14. National Sleep Foundation (n.d.). Lack of sleep is affecting Americans, finds the National Sleep Foundation. Retrieved from National Sleep Foundation: https://sleepfoundation.org/media-center/press-release/lack-sleep-affecting-americans-finds-the-national-sleep-foundation

15. National Sleep Foundation (2016). Sleep hygiene. Retrieved from National Sleep Foundation: https://sleepfoundation.org/ask-the-expert/sleep-hygiene.

16. O'shea C (2015, February 25). 8 Common and terrible sleep disorders. Retrieved from Fast Company: www.fastcompany.com/3042747/8-common-and-terrible-sleep-disorders

17. Otte JL, Davis L, Carpenter JS, Krier C, Skaar TC, Rand KL, Weaver M, Landis C, Chernyak Y, and Manchanda S (2016). Sleep disorder in breast cancer survivors. Support Care in Cancer, 24(10):4197-4205.

18. Pagel J (2007). Sleep disorders in primary care evidence-based clinical practice. In: JE Pagel, SR Pandi-Perumal, (Eds.). Primary Care Sleep Medicine. Totowa: (pp. 1-13). Totowa: Humana Press, 1-13.

19. PSQI (n.d.). Pittsburgh Sleep Questionnaire Index. Retrieved from PSQI: http://uacc. arizona.edu/sites/default/files/psqi_sleep_questionnaire_1_pg.pdf

20. Senthilvel E, Auckley D, and Dasarathy J (2011). Evaluation of sleep disorders in the primary care setting: History taking compared to questionnaires. Journal of Clinical Sleep Medicine, 7(1):41-48.

21. Siebern S, Suh S, and Nowakowski S (2012). Non-pharmacological treatment of insomnia. Neurotherapeutics, 9(4):717-727.

22. Sinha B (2009, November 22nd). Factors Affecting Sleep. Retrieved from Scribd: www. scribd.com/doc/22904067/Factors-Affecting-Sleep-The-Quality-and-Quantity-of-Sleep-Are

23. Sutter Health Palo Alto Medical Foundation (n.d.). Short- and long-term effects of sleep deprivation. Retrieved August 31, 2016, from Sutter Health , Palo Alto Medical Foundation: http://www.pamf.org/sleep/about/healtheffects.html#short

THE VALUE OF EXERCISE FOR THE BREAST CANCER SURVIVOR

Po-Ju Lin, Ph.D., M.P.H., R.D. and
Karen M. Mustian, Ph.D., M.P.H.

Breast cancer is the most commonly diagnosed cancer in women. One in eight women in the United States will be diagnosed with breast cancer in her lifetime, and the risk of getting breast cancer increases with age. In 2017, 80% of new female breast cancer patients were estimated to be 50 years old or older (American Cancer Society, 2017). Some cancer treatment-related toxicities are identical to menopausal symptoms, including hot flashes, night sweats, sleep disturbance, anxiety, depression, fatigue, bone loss, and joint and muscle pain. This is because some cancer treatments induce menopausal symptoms, and because menopause and breast cancer diagnosis might coincidentally co-occur. For example, hormonal therapy (e.g., aromatase inhibitors, tamoxifen) may cause hot flashes and musculoskeletal symptoms. Chemotherapy is associated with sleep disturbance, cognitive impairment, fatigue, and neuropathy. Surgery may cause pain, lymphedema, and limited range of motion and function of the arm. Radiation therapy may produce pain, lymphedema, and skin damage (Crandall 2004).

Both menopause symptoms and cancer treatment-related side effects may dramatically affect patients' daily activities and quality of life. Hormone (estrogen and/or progestogen) replacement therapy is known widely as an effective therapy for alleviating menopause symptoms. However, physicians often are reluctant to prescribe hormone replacement therapy to women with breast cancer and survivors, or they may prescribe it in lower doses, because it has been linked to a recurrence of breast cancer.

Physical activity, on the other hand, has shown positive effects on menopause symptoms and cancer treatment-related toxicities without additional negative side effects. Several longitudinal studies reported that menopausal women who exercise daily experience less frequent hot flashes, while women who are inactive or engage in only limited amounts of physical activity experience more vasomotor symptoms, hot flashes, and night sweats (Guthrie, 1994; Ivarsson, 1998; Ivarsson,

1998; and Gold, 2000). Seven randomized controlled trials showed that 50 to 60 minutes of walking three to four times per week at a moderate intensity for three to six months can improve hot flashes, night sweats, mood swings, and depression in menopausal women (Astrand, 2004; Elavsky, 2007; Hanachi, 2008; Lindh- Luoto, 2012; Mansikkamaki, 2012; Moilanen, 2012; and Sternfeld, 2014). Other studies showed that menopausal women, with or without breast cancer, who participated in yoga over four to 12 weeks, particularly Hatha-based (e.g., Iyengar, Tibetan, and Anusara) and restorative yoga of 60 to 120 minutes per session, one to three times per week at low to moderate intensity, reported less frequency and lower severity of hot flashes and night sweats (Elavsky, 2007; Carson, 2009; and Newton, 2014) as well as improved sleep disturbance (Chattha, 2008a; Chattha, 2008b; Mustian, 2013a; and Mustian 2013b; Newton, 2014; and Lin, 2018).

Figure 1. What is Yoga? (Mustian, 2013)

The word yoga is derived from its Sanskrit root yui, which means join together. Yoga is a practice that joins the mind and the body.

The earliest forms of yoga were rooted firmly in breathing and meditative practices. These two essential components, breathing and meditation, and an added component, physical alignment posture, form the basis and most common form of yoga practice today.

Hatha yoga, the foundation of all yoga styles, is the most popular style accepted and is practiced in Western culture. Iyengar, Anusara, and Tibetan yoga all are considered as Hatha-based yoga styles.

A Hatha yoga class usually starts with a guided meditation (e.g., body scan, calm aiding meditation), followed by breathing exercises (e.g., alternate nostril breathing, diaphragmatic breathing, vase breathing), a sequence of physical postures (e.g., child pose, cobra pose, corpse, crocodile, fish, forward bend, health bridge, half twist, shoulder stand, staff pose, sun salutation), and ends with guided relaxation in the corpse pose.

Iyengar yoga focuses on physical alignment, muscular strength and endurance, flexibility and balance, as well as concentration and meditation. Different props such as blankets, bolsters, blocks, and straps are encouraged to modify postures to meet participants' physical needs and abilities.

Restorative yoga focuses on full relaxation and is part of the Iyengar style. A restorative yoga class typically involves gentle poses, (e.g., seated forward folds, gentle backbends), light twists/stretching poses supported with props (e.g., bolsters, straps, blocks, blankets).

Physical activity also is associated with improving psychologic distress. Menopausal women who are habitual aerobic exercisers and who spend approximately 60 minutes per day on walking, cycling, or gardening have shown improved mood, depression, anxiety, and psychologic functioning. Supervised exercise is recommended particularly for women with breast cancer to improve physical, psychologic, and functional well-being after chemotherapy (Knobf, 2016). Breast cancer patients also can practice Hatha-based yoga, performed in 20- to 90-minute sessions, one to two times per week, for three to 12 weeks, to alleviate psychologic distress (Lin, 2013, and Cramer, 2018).

Weight gain is common in women at menopause (Davis, 2012). A study showed that fat mass and waist circumference were increased during the menopausal transition in women. Physical inactivity and declined estrogen are likely to be the major causes of menopausal weight gain. Walking is a safe and feasible aerobic exercise to control body weight. Seven studies showed that postmenopausal women who participated in walking, 20 to 60 minutes per day, three to five days per week at moderate intensity (45% to 69% maximal aerobic power) for three to 12 months lost more weight, reduced more body fat, and saw a greater reduction in body mass index (BMI) than those who were inactive (Martin, 1993; Brooke-Wavell, 1997; Asikainen, 2002a; Asikainen, 2002b; Wu, 2006; Ma, 2013; Zhang, 2014; and Gao, 2016).

Menopausal women who walk 30 minutes, greater than or equal to three times per week or who exercise 60 minutes daily at moderate intensity over 12 weeks, reported improved fatigue and physical menopausal symptoms (Zhang, 2014, and Kim, 2017). A supervised exercise program of aerobics alone or with resistance training is recommended for breast cancer patients, even with lymphedema, for alleviating cancer-related fatigue (Dieli-Conwright, 2014; Meneses-Echavez, 2015; and Mustian, 2017a).

A supervised exercise program usually starts with five to ten minutes of warm-up, followed by aerobic exercises like walking or ergometer-cycling alone or with strength exercises (e.g., chest and leg curls), and ends with five to ten minutes of cool-down stretching or relaxation. Studies have shown that an exercise program with just aerobic exercise or with resistance training for 20 to 60 minutes per session, one to four sessions per week at moderate intensity (50% to 80% maximal heart rate) can reduce menopausal and cancer treatment-related fatigue. This positive impact on fatigue is greater with increasing duration, frequency, and length of the exercise program (Dieli-Conwright, 2014; Meneses-Echavez, 2015; and Mustian, 2017a). Hatha, Anusara, and Iyengar yoga can help reduce fatigue and improve physical function and overall quality of life as well. Studies have demonstrated that a 60- to 90-minute yoga session, one to three times per week, for four to 12 weeks in breast cancer patients, is effective in improving fatigue (Moadel, 2007; Mustian, 2013b; Taso, 2014; Kiecolt-Glaser, 2014; Chandwani, 2014; Palesh, 2017; and Lin, 2018).

Menopausal women and women with breast cancer have a higher risk of fracture and bone loss. Bone loss occurs during the menopausal transition and also as a result of breast cancer treatments. Regular participation in weight-bearing exercise is good for skeletal health and lowering fracture risk. Combined aerobic exercise and resistance training was found to be beneficial at the skeletal site in postmenopausal women without cancer (Moreira, 2014).

Menopausal women with breast cancer should work with qualified health professionals to use the American College of Sports Medicine (ACSM) Exercise Guidelines to Preserve Bone Health during Adulthood in the General Female Population (Table1). Exercise professionals should evaluate patients' disease status, symptom burdens, physical functions, and fitness levels prior to providing exercise prescriptions to postmenopausal women or women with breast cancer.

Table 1. The American College of Sports Medicine Exercise Guidelines to Preserve Bone Health during Adulthood in the General Female Population. (Shaw, 2001, and Kohrt, 2004)

Exercise Parameters	Description
Type	Weight-bearing endurance activities (tennis, stair climbing, jogging at least intermittently during walking) and activities that involve jumping (volleyball, basketball)
Time	30 to 60 minutes per day of a combination of weight-bearing endurance activities, activities that involve jumping, and resistance exercise
Frequency	Weight-bearing endurance activities three to five times per week; resistance exercise two to three times per week
Intensity	Moderate to high intensity in terms of bone-loading forces (ground reaction forces greater than two times body weight) targeting all major muscle groups

Women who are menopausal and who have breast cancer have a greater risk of bone loss and falling than menopausal women without a history of cancer (Peppone, 2014; Chen, 2009; and Chen, 2005). Therefore, the ACSM recommends screening for fracture risk prior to exercise testing or training for women with breast cancer. Supervised exercise programs include both moderate to vigorous resistance exercise targeting the lower body, and balance exercises are recommended for menopausal women with breast cancer to preserve bone mass, maintain balance, and prevent falls (Shaw, 2001; Kohrt, 2004; Winters-Stone, 2011; Winters-Stone, 2012a; Winters-Stone, 2012b; and Winters-Stone, 2013).

The very first message that oncologists and health professionals recommend to breast cancer patients is to return to their normal daily activities and exercise routines as soon as they are able to after surgery or during and after non-surgical treatments. The ACSM recommends that cancer patients and survivors engage in 150 minutes of moderate-intensity or 75 minutes of vigorous-intensity aerobic exercise weekly, resistance training engaging all major muscle groups two to three times per week, and stretching exercises on exercising days (Table 2).

Table 2. The American College of Sports Medicine Weekly Exercise Guidelines for Individuals with Cancer (Schmitz, 2010, and ACSM, 2018)

Exercise	Aerobic Exercise	Resistance Exercise	Flexibility
Type	Prolonged and rhythmic activities engage large muscle groups (e.g., walking, cycling, and swimming)	Weight-bearing functional (e.g., sit-to-stand), free weights, or resistance machines exercises targeting all major muscle groups	Stretching for all major muscle groups; specifically to joint or muscle restriction that have resulted from cancer treatments
Time	150 minutes of moderate intensity or 75 minutes of vigorous intensity activity or an equivalent combination of the two	Greater than or equal to one set of 8 to 12 repetitions	10 to 30 seconds, hold for static stretching
Frequency	Three to five days a week	Two to three days a week	Greater than or equal to two to three days a week, with daily being most effective
Intensity	Moderate to vigorous	Start low and progress slow	Move through range of motion as tolerated

Postmenopausal women and women with breast cancer who have never engaged in any exercise program or who have never practiced yoga may need direction on how, where, and which exercise and/or yoga program to do. In addition, even if a woman has been active all her life, she still may have questions and concerns about how to exercise safely with a cancer diagnosis. Breast cancer patients should discuss their past physical activity participations and current physical activity interests with oncologists and primary care clinicians. Healthcare providers also can refer patients to qualified exercise professionals and yoga instructors before patients start a new exercise/yoga program. A qualified exercise professional should be trained and certified with the ACSM and/or American Cancer Society (ACS) as a cancer exercise trainer or clinical exercise physiologist who has considerable experience working with cancer patients and individuals 50 years old or older. A qualified yoga instructor should be certified by Yoga Alliance, have knowledge of cancer treatment-related toxicities, and have experience working with cancer patients and survivors. It is very important that patients work with primary care providers, qualified exercise professionals, and/or yoga instructors to identify risks and address potential contraindications that may affect the safety and tolerance of an exercise and/or yoga program.

Qualified exercise professionals can use this simple 5-A (Ask, Advice, Assess, Assist, and Arrange) model (Mustian, 2017b) to test, evaluate, and create an individualized exercise program for women experiencing menopausal symptoms and cancer treatment-related toxicities.

1. Ask: Do you exercise regularly? Are you currently engaging in an exercise program?

2. Advice: Review the benefits of exercise; introduce ACSM weekly exercise recommendations for cancer patients (Table 2) (Schmitz, 2010, and ACSM, 2018). If patients already are regular exercisers, ask the type, time, frequency, and intensity of the exercises they are doing.

3. Assess: If patients do not exercise regularly, review patients' medical records to see if additional medical clearance is required before performing exercise testing or starting an exercise training. Questions and concerns below need to be evaluated.

    •   Does the patient have a chronic disease such as cardiopulmonary, metabolic, or renal disease?

    •   Does the patient have signs and symptoms at rest or during usual activity (e.g., pain or discomfort in the chest, neck, jaw, arms, or other areas; shortness of breath; dizziness or syncope; orthopnea or paroxysmal nocturnal dyspnea; ankle edema; palpitations or tachycardia; intermittent claudication; heart murmur; unusual fatigue)?

    •   Does the patient have any known chronic disease, or does the patient show any signs and symptoms regardless of disease status? Additional medical clearance is required.

- For breast cancer patients with lymphedema, evaluation for arm/shoulder morbidity, function, and range of motion are recommended prior to upper body exercise (Shmitz, 2010, and ACSM, 2018).

- For breast cancer patients on hormone therapy, particularly aromatase inhibitors, pre-exercise evaluation for fracture risk is strongly recommended (Shmitz, 2010, and ACSM, 2018).

4. Assist: Create individualized exercise prescriptions based on a patient's health status, disease trajectory, previous and/or current treatment, menopause and cancer-related symptom burden, current physical function and fitness level, past and present exercise participation, and individual preferences. Encourage participation in supervised exercise programs; set appropriate short- and long-term goals; start low and progress slowly toward the ACSM exercise recommendation; identify exercise barriers and strategies to overcome them; and manage limitations, contraindications, and risks.

5. Arrange: Closely follow up with patients to evaluate disease symptoms and exercise progress; make modifications; and consult with oncologists or care providers if necessary.

Clinical evidence also has shown that participating in a low- to moderate-intensity yoga program based on Hatha, Iyangar, or Restorative yoga can improve menopause symptoms in menopausal women, with or without breast cancer. Patients who would like to try yoga should choose a yoga program led by a qualified yoga instructor who has knowledge of menopausal and cancer treatment-related side effects and who can provide necessary modifications to meet patients' physical abilities, fitness level, and range of motion (Lin, 2018). Oncologists and healthcare providers can provide appropriate referral resources to patients to help choose a safe and effective yoga program.

In conclusion, women who experience menopausal symptoms and cancer treatment-related toxicities are encouraged to participate in a supervised aerobic exercise program, with or without resistance training, to help alleviate hot flashes, night sweats, mood swings, psychologic distress, and fatigue, and reduce the risks of bone loss and fracture. Hatha-based and restorative yoga also can be considered to improve menopausal symptoms and cancer treatment-related toxicities in women with breast cancer. Patients, healthcare providers, and exercise professionals should work together to help patients to choose a safe, feasible, and effective exercise and/ or yoga program to start with and encourage them to stay physically active.

REFERENCES

1. American Cancer Society (2017). Breast Cancer Facts & Figures 2017-2018. Atlanta: American Cancer Society.

2. American College of Sports Medicine (2018). ACSM's Guidelines ror Exercise Testing and Prescription. Philadelphia: Wolters Kluwer.

3. Asikainen TM, Miilunpalo S, Oja P, Rinne M, Pasanen M, Uusi-Rasi K, and Vuori I (2002a). Randomised, controlled walking trials in postmenopausal women: The minimum dose to improve aerobic fitness? British Journal of Sports Medicine, 36(3):189-194.

4. Asikainen TM, Miilunpalo S, Oja P, Rinne M, Pasanen M, and Vuori I (2002b). Walking trials in postmenopausal women: Effect of one vs two daily bouts on aerobic fitness. Scandinavian Journal of Medicine and Science In Sports, 12(2):99-105.

5. Brooke-Wavell K, Jones PR, and Hardman AE . Brisk walking reduces calcaneal bone loss in post-menopausal women (1997). Clinical science (London, England : 1979), 92(1):75-80.

6. Carson JW, Carson KM, Porter LS, Keefe FJ, and Seewaldt VL (2009). Yoga of Awareness program for menopausal symptoms in breast cancer survivors: Results from a randomized trial. Supportive Care in Cancer: Official Journal of the Multinational Association of Supportive Care in Cancer, 17(10):1301-1309.

7. Chandwani KD, Perkins G, Nagendra HR, Raghuram NV, Spelman A, Nagarathna R, Johnson K, Fortier A, Arun B, Wei Q, Kirschbaum C, Haddad R, Morris GS, Scheetz J, Chaoul A, and Cohen L (2014). Randomized, controlled trial of yoga in women with breast cancer undergoing radiotherapy. Journal of Clinical Oncology: Official Journal of the American Society of Clinical Oncology, 32(10):1058-1065.

8. Chattha R, Nagarathna R, Padmalatha V, and Nagendra HR (2008a). Effect of yoga on cognitive functions in climacteric syndrome: A randomised control study. BJOG: An International Journal of Obstetrics and Gynaecology, 115(8):991-1000.

9. Chattha R, Raghuram N, Venkatram P, and Hongasandra NR (2008b). Treating the climacteric symptoms in Indian women with an integrated approach to yoga therapy: A randomized control study. Menopause (New York, NY), 15(5):862-870.

10. Chen Z, Maricic M, Bassford TL, Pettinger M, Ritenbaugh C, Lopez AM, Barad DH, Gass M, and Leboff MS (2005). Fracture risk among breast cancer survivors: Results From the women's health initiative observational study. Archives of Internal Medicine,

165(5):552–558.

11. Chen Z, Maricic M, Aragaki AK, Mouton C, Arendell L, Lopez AM, Bassford T, and Chlebowski RT (2009). Fracture risk increases after diagnosis of breast or other cancers in postmenopausal women: Results from the Women's Health Initiative. Osteoporosis International, 20(4):527-536.

12. Cramer H, Peng W, and Lauche R (2018). Yoga for menopausal symptoms-A systematic review and meta-analysis. Maturitas, 109:13-25.

13. Crandall C, Petersen L, Ganz PA, and Greendale GA (2004). Association of breast cancer and its therapy with menopause-related symptoms. Menopause (New York, NY), 11(5):519-530.

14. Davis SR, Castelo-Branco C, Chedraui P, Lumsden MA, Nappi RE, Shah D, and Villaseca P (2012). Understanding weight gain at menopause. Climacteric: The Journal of the International Menopause Society, 15(5):419-429.

15. Di Donato P, Giulini NA, Bacchi Modena A, et al. (2005). Factors associated with climacteric symptoms in women around menopause attending menopause clinics in Italy. Maturitas, 52(3-4):181-189.

16. D Dieli-Conwright CM, Mortimer JE, Schroeder ET, Courneya K, Demark-Wahnefried W, Buchanan TA, Tripathy D, and Bernstein L (2014). Randomized controlled trial to evaluate the effects of combined progressive exercise on metabolic syndrome in breast cancer survivors: Rationale, design, and methods. BMC cancer, 14:238.

17. Elavsky S and McAuley E (2007). Physical activity and mental health outcomes during menopause: A randomized controlled trial. Annals of Behavioral Medicine: A Publication of the Society of Behavioral Medicine, 33(2):132-142.

18. Gao HL, Gao HX, Sun FM, and Zhang L (2016). Effects of walking on body composition in perimenopausal and postmenopausal women: A systematic review and meta-analysis. Menopause (New York, NY), 23(8):928-934.

19. Gold EB, Sternfeld B, Kelsey JL, Brown C, Mouton C, Reame N, Salamone L, and Stellato R (2000). Relation of demographic and lifestyle factors to symptoms in a multi-racial/ethnic population of women 40-55 years of age. American journal of epidemiology, 152(5):463-473.

20. Guthrie JR, Smith AM, Dennerstein L, and Morse C (1994). Physical activity and the menopause experience: A cross-sectional study. Maturitas, 20(2-3):71-80.

21. Hanachi PaG and Golkho S (2008). Assessment of Soy Phytoestrogens and exercise on lipid profiles and menopause symptoms in menopausal women. Journal of Biological Sciences, 8(4):789-793.

22. Ivarsson T, Spetz AC, and Hammar M (1998). Physical exercise and vasomotor symptoms in postmenopausal women. Maturitas, 29(2):139-146.

23. Kiecolt-Glaser JK, Bennett JM, Andridge R, Peng J, Shapiro CL, Malarkey WB, Emery CF, Layman R, Mrozek EE, and Glaser R (2014). Yoga's impact on inflammation, mood,

and fatigue in breast cancer survivors: A randomized controlled trial. Journal of clinical oncology : official journal of the American Society of Clinical Oncology, 32(10):1040-1049.

24. Kim TH, Chang JS, Park KS, Park J, Kim N, Lee JI, andKong ID (2017). Effects of exercise training on circulating levels of Dickkpof-1 and secreted frizzled-related protein-1 in breast cancer survivors: A pilot single-blind randomized controlled trial. PloS one, 12(2):e0171771.

25. Knobf MT, Jeon S, Smith B, Harris L, Kerstetter J, Thompson AS, and Insogna K (2016). Effect of a randomized controlled exercise trial on bone outcomes: Influence of adjuvant endocrine therapy. Breast cancer research and treatment, 155(3):491-500.

26. Kohrt WM, Bloomfield SA, Little KD, Nelson ME, and Yingling VR (2004). American College of Sports Medicine Position Stand: Physical activity and bone health. Medicine and Science in Sports and Exercise, 36(11):1985-1996.

27. Lin PJ, Peppone LJ, Janelsins MC, Mohile SG, Kamen CS, Kleckner IR, Fung C, Asare M, Cole CL, Culakova E, and Mustian KM (2018). Yoga for the management of cancer treatment-related toxicities. Current Oncology Reports, 20(1):5.

28. Lindh-Astrand L, Nedstrand E, Wyon Y, and Hammar M (2004). Vasomotor symptoms and quality of life in previously sedentary postmenopausal women randomised to physical activity or estrogen therapy. Maturitas, 48(2):97-105.

29. Luoto R, Moilanen J, Heinonen R, Mikkola T, Raitanen J, Tomas E, Ojala K, Mansikkamäki K, and Nygård CH (2012). Effect of aerobic training on hot flushes and quality of life--a randomized controlled trial. Annals of Medicine, 44(6):616-626.

30. Ma D, Wu L, and He Z (2013). Effects of walking on the preservation of bone mineral density in perimenopausal and postmenopausal women: A systematic review and meta-analysis. Menopause (New York, NY), 20(11):1216-1226.

31. Mansikkamäki K, Raitanen J, Nygård CH, Heinonen R, Mikkola T, EijaTomás, and Luoto R (2012). Sleep quality and aerobic training among menopausal women--a randomized controlled trial. Maturitas, 72(4):339-345.

32. Martin D and Notelovitz M (1993). Effects of aerobic training on bone mineral density of postmenopausal women. Journal of Bone and Mineral Research: The Official Journal of the American Society for Bone and Mineral Research, 8(8):931-936.

33. Meneses-Echavez JF, Gonzalez-Jimenez E, and Ramirez-Velez R (2015). Effects of supervised exercise on cancer-related fatigue in breast cancer survivors: A systematic review and meta-analysis. BMC Cancer, 15:77.

34. Moadel AB, Shah C, Wylie-Rosett J, Harris MS, Patel SR, Hall CB, and Sparano JA (2007). Randomized controlled trial of yoga among a multiethnic sample of breast cancer patients: Effects on quality of life. Journal of Clinical Oncology: Official Journal of the American Society of Clinical Oncology, 25(28):4387-4395.

35. Moilanen JM, Mikkola TS, Raitanen JA, Heinonen RH, Tomas EI, Nygård CH, and Luoto RM (2012). Effect of aerobic training on menopausal symptoms--a randomized controlled trial. Menopause (New York, NY), 19(6):691-696.

36. Moreira LD, Oliveira ML, Lirani-Galvao AP, Marin-Mio RV, Santos RN, and Lazaretti-Castro M (2014). Physical exercise and osteoporosis: Effects of different types of exercises on bone and physical function of postmenopausal women. Arquivos Brasileiros de Endocrinologia e Metabologia, 58(5):514-522.

37. Mustian KM (2013a). Yoga as treatment for insomnia among cancer patients and survivors: A systematic review. European Medical Journal. Oncology, 1:106-115.

38. Mustian KM, Sprod LK, Janelsins M, Peppone LJ, Palesh OG, Chandwani K, Reddy PS, Melnik MK, Heckler C, and Morrow GR (2013b). Multicenter, randomized controlled trial of yoga for sleep quality among cancer survivors. Journal of Clinical Oncology: Official Journal of the American Society of Clinical Oncology, 31(26):3233-3241.

39. Mustian KM, Alfano CM, Heckler C, Kleckner AS, Kleckner IR, Leach CR, Mohr D, Palesh OG, Peppone LJ, Piper BF, Scarpato J, Smith T, Sprod LK, and Miller SM (2017a). Comparison of pharmaceutical, psychological, and exercise treatments for cancer-related fatigue: A meta-analysis. JAMA oncology, 3(7):961-968.

40. Mustian K, Lin P, Cole C, Loh KP, and Magnuson A (2017b). Exercise and the older cancer survivor. In: Geriatric Oncology. New York: Springer, 1-22.

41. Newton KM, Reed SD, Guthrie KA, Sherman KJ, Booth-LaForce C, Caan B, Sternfeld B, Carpenter JS, Learman LA, Freeman EW, Cohen LS, Joffe H, Anderson GL, Larson JC, Hunt JR, Ensrud KE, and LaCroix AZ (2014). Efficacy of yoga for vasomotor symptoms: A randomized controlled trial. Menopause (New York, NY), 21(4):339-346.

42. Palesh O, Scheiber C, Kesler S, Mustian K, Koopman C, and Schapira L (2017). Management of side effects during and post-treatment in breast cancer survivors. The Breast Journal, 20(2):167-175.

43. Peppone LJ, Mustian KM, Rosier RN, et al. Bone health issues in breast cancer survivors: A Medicare Current Beneficiary Survey (MCBS) study. Supportive Care in Cancer. 2014;22(1):245-51.

44. Schmitz KH, Courneya KS, Matthews C, Demark-Wahnefried W, Galvão DA, Pinto BM, Irwin ML, Wolin KY, Segal RJ, Lucia A, Schneider CM, von Gruenigen VE, and Schwartz AL (2010). American College of Sports Medicine roundtable on exercise guidelines for cancer survivors. Medicine and Science in Sports and Exercise, 42(7):1409-1426.

45. Shaw JM, Witzke KA, and Winters KM (2001). Exercise for Skeletal Health and Osteoporosis Prevention, ACSM Resource Manual. Philadelphia: Williams & Wilkins Publishers.

46. Sternfeld B, Guthrie KA, Ensrud KE, LaCroix AZ, Larson JC, Dunn AL, Anderson GL, Seguin RA, Carpenter JS, Newton KM, Reed SD, Freeman EW, Cohen LS, Joffe H, Roberts M, and Caan BJ (2014). Efficacy of exercise for menopausal symptoms: A randomized controlled trial. Menopause (New York, NY), 21(4):330-338.

47. Taso CJ, Lin HS, Lin WL, Chen SM, Huang WT, and Chen SW (2014). The effect of yoga exercise on improving depression, anxiety, and fatigue in women with breast cancer: A randomized controlled trial. The Journal of Nursing Research: JNR, 22(3):155-164.

48. Winters-Stone KM, Dobek J, Nail L, Bennett JA, Leo MC, Naik A, and Schwartz A (2011). Strength training stops bone loss and builds muscle in postmenopausal breast cancer survivors: A randomized, controlled trial. Breast Cancer Research and Treatment, 127(2):447-456.

49. Winters-Stone KM, Dobek J, Bennett JA, Nail LM, Leo MC, and Schwartz A (2012a). The effect of resistance training on muscle strength and physical function in older, postmenopausal breast cancer survivors: A randomized controlled trial. Journal of Cancer Survivorship: Research and Practice, 6(2):189-199.

50. Winters-Stone KM, Leo MC, and Schwartz A (2012b). Exercise effects on hip bone mineral density in older, post-menopausal breast cancer survivors are age dependent. Archives of Osteoporosis, 7:301-306.

51. Winters-Stone KM, Dobek J, Nail LM, Bennett JA, Leo MC, Torgrimson-Ojerio B, Luoh SW, and Schwartz A (2013). Impact + resistance training improves bone health and body composition in prematurely menopausal breast cancer survivors: A randomized controlled trial. Osteoporosis international: A Journal Established as a Result of Cooperation Between the European Foundation for Osteoporosis and the National Osteoporosis Foundation of the USA, 24(5):1637-1646.

52. Wu J, Oka J, Higuchi M, Tabata I, Toda T, Fujioka M, Fuku N, Teramoto T, Okuhira T, Ueno T, Uchiyama S, Urata K, Yamada K, and Ishimi Y (2006). Cooperative effects of isoflavones and exercise on bone and lipid metabolism in postmenopausal Japanese women: A randomized placebo-controlled trial. Metabolism: Clinical and Experimental, 55(4):423-433.

53. Zhang J, Chen G, Lu W, Yan X, Zhu S, Dai Y, Xi S, Yao C, and Bai W (2014). Effects of physical exercise on health-related quality of life and blood lipids in perimenopausal women: A randomized placebo-controlled trial. Menopause (New York, NY), 21(12):1269-1276.

FERTILITY AND PREGNANCY IN YOUNG WOMEN WITH BREAST CANCER CARE

Wendy S. Vitek, M.D.

Approximately 7% of women with breast cancer are diagnosed prior to age 40 (Howlader, 2011). Fertility and pregnancy are concerns for approximately half of young women diagnosed with breast cancer (Letourneau, 2012, and Ruddy, 2014) and many will face premature ovarian insufficiency and infertility as a consequence of chemotherapy and endocrine therapy. These important concerns can impact quality of life as well as treatment decisions, adherence to endocrine therapy, and possibly survival (Llarena, 2015). As a result, fertility counseling is an important aspect of comprehensive cancer care for young women with breast cancer. Options for optimizing fertility include fertility preservation prior to chemotherapy, ovarian protection during chemotherapy, and fertility treatment after endocrine therapy. Pregnancy after breast cancer appears to be a safe option. Pregnancy through a gestational carrier, however, is an alternative.

Fertility Preservation Prior to Cancer Therapy

Chemotherapy can lead to infertility by reducing ovarian reserve. Ovarian reserve reflects the pool of primordial follicles from which an oocyte is selected for ovulation. The ovarian reserve declines with age, and menopause occurs when the ovarian reserve is nearly exhausted. Alkylating agents, such as cyclophosphamide, can accelerate the loss of primordial follicles by inducing double-strand DNA breaks and apoptosis (Bedoschi, 2016). As a result, 26% to 77% of young women with breast cancer who are treated with cyclophosphamide will develop chemotherapy-induced amenorrhea and are at risk for early menopause (Zavos, 2016). Factors associated with chemotherapy-induced amenorrhea include high-dose cyclophosphamide therapy, advanced reproductive age at the time of chemotherapy, diminished ovarian reserve prior to chemotherapy, and prolonged use of endocrine therapy, such as tamoxifen.

Given the increased risk of infertility after breast cancer therapy, oocyte, embryo, and ovarian tissue cryopreservation can be performed prior to neoadjuvant or adjuvant chemotherapy to preserve fertility. Oocyte and embryo banking require controlled ovarian hyperstimulation and oocyte retrieval, while ovarian tissue cryopreservation requires a laparoscopic partial or complete oophorectomy. Timing, safety, success rates, and cost factor into the decision to pursue these options.

Advances in ovarian hyperstimulation protocols allow for oocyte and embryo banking to be accomplished within two weeks of a fertility preservation consultation. Conventional ovarian hyperstimulation protocols start in the early follicular phase of the menstrual cycle requiring two to six weeks to complete oocyte or embryo banking, depending on the phase of the menstrual cycle during which the patient presents. Random-start ovarian hyperstimulation protocols, however, start in the late follicular phase and luteal phase of the menstrual cycle and appear to have comparable outcomes to the conventional protocols that start in the early follicular phase (Cakmak, 2013). Random-start ovarian hyperstimulation protocols reduce the time to complete oocyte or embryo banking to two weeks and avoid delaying the initiation of chemotherapy. Adjuvant chemotherapy typically follows surgery and recovery. One or two banking cycles can be performed during the typical four-week, post-surgical recovery period without delaying the start of chemotherapy (Baynosa, 2009, and Letourneau, 2017). Neoadjuvant chemotherapy typically starts two to three weeks after the diagnosis and prior to surgery, given the need to complete the evaluation and formulate the treatment plan, and for the patient to understand her diagnosis and options. A two-week window for oocyte or embryo banking exists, even in the case of neoadjuvant chemotherapy. Ovarian tissue cryopreservation is an alternative option for women who cannot delay the start of chemotherapy by two weeks. Laparoscopic partial or complete oophorectomy for ovarian tissue cryopreservation can be performed at the time of port placement to minimize cost and anesthetic risks.

Safety of oocyte, embryo, and ovarian tissue banking is a top concern of patients and providers. Supra-physiologic estradiol and progesterone levels encountered during and after controlled ovarian hyperstimulation for oocyte or embryo banking can be a concern for women with hormone sensitive breast cancers, and care should be taken to minimize estradiol levels during treatment. Several adjustments can be made to conventional and random-start ovarian hyperstimulation protocols to minimize estradiol and progesterone levels in women with hormone sensitive breast cancers. Letrozole, an aromatase inhibitor, can be taken during controlled ovarian hyperstimulation and immediately after oocyte retrieval to lower estradiol levels. This approach results in a similar number of oocytes and embryos banked when compared to controlled ovarian hyperstimulation without letrozole and significantly lowers peak serum estradiol levels among women treated with letrozole (Oktay, 2006). The safety of letrozole ovarian hyperstimulation protocols has been examined in a study comparing 79 breast cancer patients, 81% of whom had an estrogen-receptor positive cancer, with 136 control patients who did not undergo ovarian stimulation. The median follow-up time of the study was two years, ranging from 23 months in the letrozole group to 33 months in the control group. During this time period, there were three (4%) recurrences in the letrozole group and 11 (8%) in the control group. There was no significant difference in relapse-free survival between the groups. This study was not randomized, so selection bias is possible, but the experimental and control groups were similar with respect to age and prognostic markers for cancer recurrence. Long-term, follow-up data are not yet available, although recurrence risk generally is thought to be highest during the first two years after treatment (Azim, 2008).

Another adjustment to minimize peak estradiol and progesterone levels is to utilize a gonadotropin-releasing hormone (GnRH) agonist to induce final oocyte maturation in preparation for oocyte retrieval instead of a standard human chorionic gonadotropin (HCG) trigger (Anderson, 1999). A GnRH agonist triggers a leuteinizing hormone (LH) surge, but does not support sustained release of LH in the luteal phase. The lack of LH support induces lysis of the multiple corpus luteums that are a consequence of controlled ovarian hyperstimulation. Leuteolysis leads to a rapid decline in estradiol and progesterone levels post retrieval, which minimizes supra-physiologic hormone exposure in women with hormone-sensitive breast cancers without compromising the number or quality of oocytes or embryos banked. This approach also nearly eliminates the risk of ovarian hyperstimulation syndrome, which is a rare but serious complication of oocyte and embryo banking.

Ovarian tissue cryopreservation remains experimental and there are concerns regarding safety. Laparoscopic partial or complete oophorectomy can be performed at any point in the menstrual cycle and does not require controlled ovarian hyperstimulation. The cortical ovarian tissue, which is comprised of primordial follicles, is dissected into small fragments and cryopreserved.

Autotransplantation of the thawed, ovarian cortical tissue to the residual ovary or the pelvic side wall has resulted in spontaneous and in-vitro fertilization pregnancies (Donnez, 2013) among women with breast cancer and other malignancies. Although there have been no reported cases of recurrent cancer after ovarian tissue autotransplantation, there is concern that transplanted ovarian tissue could be contaminated with cancer cells, particularly in cancers such as breast cancer which can metastasize to the ovary (Bastings, 2013). In-vitro maturation of primordial follicles would avoid the need for and risks of ovarian tissue cryopreservation. This approach has been successful in animal models but has not yet produced a live birth in humans (Smitz, 2010). Mature oocyte and immature oocytes have been retrieved from ovarian tissue at the time of partial or complete oophorectomy in unstimulated patients (Prasath, 2014, and Uzela, 2015). Mature oocytes have been fertilized, and embryo cryopreservation has been performed. Immature oocytes can be matured *in vitro* using culture media treated with gonadotropins, and mature oocytes have been cryopreserved from this technique. These strategies have resulted in live births among women with ovarian cancers, which is a contraindication to controlled ovarian hyperstimulation and autotransplantation of thawed, cryopreserved ovarian tissue. While these cases demonstrate evidence that this approach can result in live birth, this option is not widely offered to women with breast cancer given that the efficiency of oocyte recovery is not known.

Success rates (defined as a live birth, after oocyte, embryo, and ovarian tissue cryopreservation preformed prior to chemotherapy among young women with breast cancer) are lacking. Women with breast cancer typically are counseled on their chance of a live birth based on their age at the time of oocyte or embryo banking, and the chance of live birth is extrapolated from women of a similar age who underwent in-vitro fertilization (IVF) for infertility-related diagnoses (Oktay, 2015). Cumulative live birth rates per oocyte retrieval from IVF and frozen embryo transfer cycles performed in the United States (U.S.) in 2014 are 54.4% for women less than 35 years of age, 42% for women age 35 to 37 years, 26.6% for women age 38 to 40 years, 13.3% for women age 41 to 42 years, and 3.9% for women greater than 42 years of age (SART, 2014). Success rates for ovarian tissue cryopreservation and subsequent autotransplantation have been reported as 57.5% live birth rate in a meta-analysis comprised of 309 cases, of which 78% had been diagnosed with a malignancy with a mean age of 29.3 years at the time of ovarian tissue cryopreservation and mean age of 33.0 years at the time of autotransplantation (Pacheco, 2017).

Women with cancer cite cost as the most significant factor in their decision about pursuing fertility preservation, as insurance coverage for oocyte, embryo, or ovarian tissue cryopreservation is rare (Walter, 2017). The average cost in the U.S. of one fertility-preservation cycle of ovarian stimulation and embryo or oocyte cryopreservation is $12,737, and the average cost of ovarian tissue cryopreservation (anecdotal) may be as high as $10,000 (medicaldaily.com, 2017). Connecticut and Rhode Island recently became the first U.S. states to pass legislation requiring private insurance coverage of fertility-preservation services for patients about to undergo a medical treatment that can impair fertility (Cardozo, 2017), although it seems unlikely that universal private insurance coverage will occur, given that most states do not mandate diagnosis and treatment of infertility.

While most breast cancers are sporadic, testing for hereditary breast and ovarian cancer often is warranted in younger women with breast cancer or those with a family history of either disease in multiple relatives. Identification of a genetic predisposition raises unique considerations for fertility. Although the prevalence is low in the general population, a majority of patients with inherited breast or ovarian cancer will carry a mutation in either BRCA 1 or BRCA 2. Reproductive age women who carry these mutations often are counseled for risk-reducing surgery, including mastectomy and bilateral salpingo-oophorectomy (BSO) to prevent occurrence of cancer. Bilateral salpingo-oophorectomy typically is recommended prior to the age at which the youngest family member was diagnosed with cancer but, ideally, after childbearing is complete. In circumstances where BSO cannot be delayed, fertility preservation is an option. Oocyte or embryo cryopreservation are the preferred options, as ovarian tissue freezing is not recommended given the potential risk of ovarian cancer with autologous transplantation. Some evidence suggests that ovarian reserve may be reduced in BRCA mutations carriers leading to a diminished response to controlled ovarian hyperstimulation (Peccatori, 2017). However, these findings are inconsistent and considered controversial. Since patients typically do not have a firm time constraint prior to risk-reducing BSO, multiple IVF cycles could be attempted to increase the total number of cryopreserved oocytes or embryos in the event of poor response. Patients who carry a BRCA mutation can consider preimplantation genetic diagnosis (PGD) as a means to screen embryos for the affected gene. Preimplantation genetic diagnosis can be done at the time of fertility preservation or at the time when embryos will be utilized for pregnancy.

Ovarian Protection during Cancer Therapy

Gonadotropin-releasing hormone agonist co-treatment during chemotherapy has been proposed for ovarian protection. As chemotherapies such as cyclophosphamide induce apoptosis of growing follicles, there will be less negative feedback by estradiol and inhibin B leading to an increase in follicle-stimulating hormone (FSH)-driven follicular recruitment and accelerated folliculogenesis. Gonadotropin-releasing hormone agonists have been hypothesized to preserve ovarian reserve through several mechanisms. Depot GnRH agonist induces downregulation of FSH production seven to ten days post administration, which leads to suppression of the hypothalamic-pituitary-ovarian axis. The lower circulating levels of FSH diminish the accelerated loss of ovarian reserve mediated by FSH-driven follicular recruitment. Another possible protective mechanism is that GnRH agonists decrease ovarian perfusion, reducing delivery of the chemotherapeutic agent to the ovaries. Goserelin and triprorelin are the GnRH agonists most often used in recent ovarian protection studies in breast cancer patients, while buserelin and leuprolide have been used in studies published in the 1980s and 1990s as well as in patients with hematologic malignancies. Side effects of GnRH agonists related to the induced hypoestrogenic state include hot flashes, vaginal dryness, and bone loss. Norethindrone acetate is a progestin with estrogenic properties and has been shown to preserve bone mass and significantly reduce vasomotor symptoms without increasing the rate of vaginal bleeding. Add-back therapy may not be appropriate in women with hormone receptor-positive breast cancer. With respect to the safety of GnRH agonist co-treatment, multiple studies have concluded that chemotherapy-induced amenorrhea results in improved disease-free and overall survival in women with breast cancer. Given the possible survival benefit associated with premature ovarian insufficiency, trials of GnRH agonists have examined disease-free and overall survival of participants to determine if ovarian protection reduces these important outcomes. In the Prevention of Early Menopause Study (POEMS), women with hormone receptor-negative early breast cancer were randomized to co-treatment with goserelin versus chemotherapy alone (Moore, 2015). Women with hormone receptor-negative early breast cancer were studied to eliminate the confounder of tamoxifen use. Despite closing the trial early due to funding issues, a reduction in premature ovarian failure was observed with goserelin co-treatment. In addition, a nonsignificant trend toward disease-free survival, as well as a significant increase in overall survival, was observed in the goserelin group, suggesting safety of GnRH agonist co-treatment in women with triple-negative cancer. A possible explanation for this finding is that LH receptors frequently are present in triple-negative cancers. Preclinical studies have shown that the use of GnRH analogs in xenograft models of triple-negative breast cancer is associated with growth inhibition, reduction in metastasis, and apoptotic cell death. It is possible that the GnRH agonist co-treatment may contribute to obtaining remission, and it does not appear that ovarian protection is harmful for disease-free women or to overall survival among women with triple-negative breast cancer.

Given the challenge of conducting research that is powered to compare and track long-term outcomes such as fertility, there are limited randomized data on fertility-related outcomes such as fecundity, miscarriage rate, and maternal and neonatal outcomes after co-treatment with a GnRH agonist during chemotherapy. As a result, most GnRH agonist co-treatment studies are designed to show a difference in the rate of resumption of menses or premature ovarian insufficiency at one to two years after chemotherapy. More recent studies have examined the endpoint of diminished ovarian reserve as measured by changes in ovarian reserve markers such as antimüllerian hormone (AMH) and antral follicle count (AFC). To date, 12 randomized controlled trials have been published on co-treatment with a GnRH agonist or chemotherapy alone in women with breast cancer. A recent meta-analysis found a significant reduction in the odds of developing premature ovarian insufficiency in women with breast cancer who were co-treated with a GnRH agonist during chemotherapy compared to women who received chemotherapy alone, with an odds ratio that favors GnRH agonist co-treatment of 0.34 and a 95% confidence interval of 0.025 to 0.46 and a P value of 0.026 (Letourneau, 2012).

Several criticisms of the individual trials and, thus, the meta-analysis exist. First, several trials enrolled women in their mid to late 40s. Given the high rates of infertility and natural menopause in this population, fertility outcomes could not be assessed directly. The chemotherapy regimens used in trials performed 20 to 30 years ago typically included higher cumulative doses of cyclophosphamide and were more ovarian toxic than current regimens that use lower cumulative doses of cyclophosphamide. This resulted in heterogeneity of the chemotherapy regimens in the meta-analysis. Several trials included women with hormone-positive cancers that typically are treated with tamoxifen after chemotherapy. Tamoxifen is a confounder, as it is associated with amenorrhea. Some studies did not provide information on hormone-positive cancers and treatment with tamoxifen. The definition of premature ovarian insufficiency varied between trials. Some studies based the diagnosis solely on patient-reported amenorrhea lasting greater than six to 12 months, whereas others included FSH values in the diagnosis. Finally, most studies were powered to show a difference in rate of premature ovarian insufficiency and not fertility outcomes. Of note, several studies were stopped prematurely because of a lack of a benefit noted at the interim analysis. Information on how participants were tracked for fertility outcomes is limited in most of the trials, thus limiting the ability to objectively assess differences in these endpoints.

Despite a possible 34% reduction in premature ovarian insufficiency in women with breast cancer who are co-treated with an GnRH agonist during chemotherapy, neither the American Society for Reproductive Medicine (ASRM) or the American Society of Clinical Oncology (ASCO) recommend GnRH agonist co-treatment as a primary means of fertility preservation, possibly due to the limited efficacy and limitations in the data (Ethics Committee of ASRM, 2013, and Loren, 2013). Both societies recommended that GnRH agonist co-treatment be offered as a means of fertility preservation in addition to, but not instead of, oocyte, embryo, or ovarian tissue cryopreservation.

Fertility Treatment after Cancer Therapy

Factors that contribute to decisions regarding fertility treatment after breast cancer thearpy include the patient's age, ovarian reserve, and duration of endocrine therapy. Advanced reproductive age is associated with diminished ovarian reserve, diminished oocyte quality, and embryo aneuploidy which contribute to miscarriage and infertility. Antimüllerian hormone is produced by the granulosa cells of preantal follicles, and the serum level reflects the ovarian reserve. Pretreatment AMH levels are predictive of long-term ovarian function with lower AMH levels associated with chemotherapy-induced amenorrhea and premature ovarian insufficiency (Dillon, 2013). In women less than 35 years of age who are treated with chemotherapy for breast cancer, AMH levels decline in the year following treatment, slightly increase two years after treatment, and little additional recovery is noted at five years posttreatment. In addition, recovery of AMH does not reach the level expected based on age. Posttreatment AMH levels may be used to estimate the length of reproductive lifespan and guide treatment decisions, although it is unclear if AMH levels predict live birth among women treated for breast cancer.

Endocrine therapy with tamoxifen in premenopausal women with hormone-sensitive breast cancer does not appear to further reduce AMH levels, although it is associated with amenorrhea and reduced childbearing (Shandley, 2017). Tamoxifen is a teratogen, and pregnancy should be avoided during treatment. Tamoxifen therapy currently is recommended for five to ten years, and this delay in childbearing can reduce ovarian reserve due to aging. Given these fertility concerns, young women with breast cancer often are reluctant to initiate tamoxifen therapy and are more likely to discontinue therapy prior to five years of treatment.

Women who bank oocytes and embryos prior to chemotherapy often will opt to proceed with a frozen embryo transfer in order to become pregnant shortly after discontinuation of tamoxifen and to utilize embryos with a lower risk of aneuploidy given that the embryos often are banked years prior to the transfer. Women with premature ovarian insufficiency who banked ovarian tissue prior to chemotherapy may opt for autotransplantation after thorough counseling regarding the possible risk of recurrent cancer. Women with hormone-sensitive cancer who did not bank oocyte, embryos, or ovarian tissue and exhibit diminished ovarian reserve may opt for superovulation with letrozole to reduce their estradiol exposure during fertility treatment, IVF, or possibly donor-egg IVF, depending on the severity of their diminished ovarian reserve. Cancer treatment prior to IVF is associated with lower responsiveness to controlled ovarian hyperstimulation and lower live birth rates (Barton, 2012). Women with breast cancer appear to have a lower chance of live birth if IVF with autologous oocytes is performed after cancer therapy, although their chance of live birth is similar to women without cancer when donor oocytes are used (Luke, 2016). For women with breast cancer who do not want to delay childbearing for the completion of tamoxifen treatment or for those with other medical contraindications, gestational surrogacy may be a suitable option.

Pregnancy after Breast Cancer

Many young women with breast cancer will fear pregnancy given concerns regarding recurrence and the effects of cancer treatment on pregnancy. Retrospective data show that pregnancy after estrogen receptor-negative and positive breast cancer is not associated with differences in disease-free and overall survival, although survivor bias may factor into these findings (Nye, 2017). Timing of conception after the disease still is a matter of debate, especially in women receiving adjuvant endocrine therapy. In general, patients are advised to delay pregnancy at least two years after diagnosis, as the risk of recurrence is highest in this time frame and to restart tamoxifen once pregnancy and lactation are complete. An ongoing prospective trial assessing safety of interrupting endocrine treatment to allow conception will provide valuable counseling information. Pregnancy after treatment for ductal carcinoma *in situ* does not appear to increase preterm births, low birth weight, or small-for-gestational-age neonates (Hartnett, 2017). Breastfeeding after surgery and radiation for breastfeeding can be challenging but should not be discouraged, as it does not appear to increase the risk of recurrence and does not pose any risk to the child. (See the chapter entitled Breastfeeding after Breast Cancer.)

CONCLUSION

Young women with breast cancer have safe and effective options for fertility preservation through modified, controlled, ovarian hyperstimulation protocols for oocyte and embryo cryopreservation, ovarian protection with GnRH agonist co-treatment during chemotherapy, ovarian reserve assessment through pre- and posttreatment Antimüllerian hormone levels, and fertility treatment such as IVF and gestational carrier after breast cancer therapy. In addition, women with BRCA mutations can bank oocytes or embryos prior to risk-reducing BSO and have the option of PGD to reduce the risk of BRCA mutation in their children. Multiple retrospective trials support that pregnancy and breastfeeding appear to be safe options for both mother and child in the case of both estrogen receptor-negative and positive disease. Future advances in comprehensive fertility care for women with breast cancer would include the ability to reliably screen ovarian tissue for metatastic cells prior to autotransplantation, in-vitro maturation of primordial follicles from ovarian tissue to achieve a live birth, evidence based guidance regarding the safety of interrupting endocrine therapy for pregnancy and lactation, and universal insurance coverage for fertility preservation and fertility treatment after cancer therapy.

REFERENCES

1. Anderson RA, Kinniburgh D, and Baird D (1999). Preliminary experience of the use of a gonadotropin-releasing hormone antagonist in ovulation induction/in-vitro fertilization prior to cancer treatment. Human Reproduction, 14(10):2665-2668.

2. Azim A, Costantini-Ferrando M, and Oktay K (2008). Safety of fertility preservation by ovarian stimulation with letrozole and gonadotropins in patients with breast cancer: A prospective controlled study. Journal of Clinical Oncology, 26(16):2630-2635.

3. Barton SE, Missmer SA, Berry KF, and Ginsburg ES (2012). Female cancer survivors are low responders and have reduced success compared with other patients undergoing assisted reproductive technologies. Fertility and Sterility, 97(2):381-386.

4. Bastings L, Beerendonk CC, Westphal JR, Massuger LF, Kaal SE, van Leeuwen FE, Braat DD, and Peek R (2013). Autotransplantation of cryopreserved ovarian tissue in cancer survivors and the risk of reintroducing malignancy: A systematic review. Human Reproduction Update, 19(5):483-506.

5. Baynosa J, Westphal LM, Madrigrano A, and Wapnir I (2009). Timing of breast cancer treatments with oocyte retrieval and embryo cryopreservation. Journal of the American College of Surgeons, 209(5):603–607.

6. Bedoschi G, Navarro PA, and Oktay K (2016). Chemotherapy-induced damage to ovary: Mechanisms and clinical impact. Future Oncology, 12(20):2333–2344.

7. Cakmak H, Katz A, Cedars MI, and Rosen MP (2013). Effective method for emergency fertility preservation: Random-start controlled ovarian stimulation. Fertility and Sterility, 100(6):1673-1680.

8. Cardozo ER, Huber WJ, Stuckey AR, and Alvero RJ (2017). Mandating coverage for fertility preservation - A step in the right direction. The New England Journal of Medicine, 377(17):1607-1609.

9. Dillon KE, Sammel MD, Prewitt M, Ginsberg JP, Walker D, Mersereau JE, Gosiengfiao Y, and Gracia CR (2013). Pretreatment antimüllerian hormone levels determine rate of posttherapy ovarian reserve recovery: Acute changes in ovarian reserve during and after chemotherapy. Fertility and Sterility, 99(2):477-483.

10. Donnez J and Dolmans MM (2013). Fertility preservation in women. Nature Reviews. Endocrinology, 9(12):735-749.

11. Ethics Committee of ASRM (2013). Fertility preservation and reproduction in patients facing gonadotoxic therapies: A committee opinion. Fertility and Sterility, 100(5):1224-1231

12. Hartnett KP, Ward KC, Kramer MR, Lash TL, Mertens AC, Spencer JB, Fothergill A, and Howards PP (2017). The risk of preterm birth and growth restriction in pregnancy after cancer. International Journal of Cancer, 141(11):2187-2196.

13. Howlader N, Noone AM, Krapcho M, Garshell J, Miller D, Altekruse SF, Kosary CL, Yu M, Ruhl J, Tatalovich Z,Mariotto A, Lewis DR, Chen HS, Feuer EJ, and Cronin KA (eds). (2014). SEER Cancer Statistics Review, 1975-2011. Bethesda, MD: National Cancer Institute.

14. Letourneau JM, Ebbel EE, Katz PP, Katz A, Ai WZ, Chien AJ, Melisko ME, Cedars MI, and Rosen MP (2012). Pretreatment fertility counseling and fertility preservation improve quality of life in reproductive age women with cancer. Cancer, 118(6):1710–1717.

15. Letourneau JM, Ebbel EE, Katz PP, Oktay KH, McCulloch CE, Ai WZ, Chien AJ, Melisko ME, Cedars MI, and Rosen MP (2012). Acute ovarian failure underestimates age-specific reproductive impairment for young women undergoing chemotherapy for cancer. Cancer, 118(7):1922-1929.

16. Letourneau JM, Sinha N, Wald K, Harris E, Quinn M, Imbar T, Mok-Lin E, Chien AJ, and Rosen M (2017). Random start ovarian stimulation for fertility preservation appears unlikely to delay initiation of neoadjuvant chemotherapy for breast cancer. Human Reproduction, 32(10):2123-2129.

17. Llarena NC, Estevez SL, Tucker SL, and Jeruss JS (2015). Impact of fertility concerns on tamoxifen initiation and persistence. Journal of the National Cancer Institute, 107(10):djv202.

18. Loren AW, Mangu PB, Beck LN, Brennan L, Magdalinski AJ, Partridge AH, Quinn G, Wallace WH, and Oktay K; American Society of Clinical Oncology (2013). Fertility preservation for patients with cancer: American Society of Clinical Oncology clinical practice guideline. Journal of Clinical Oncology, 31(19):2500-2510.

19. Luke B, Brown MB, Missmer SA, Spector LG, Leach RE, Williams M, Koch L, Smith YR, Stern JE, Ball GD, and Schymura MJ (2016). Assisted reproductive technology use and outcomes among women with a history of cancer. Human Reproduction, 31(1):183-189.

20. https://www.medicaldaily.com/why-doctors-believe-ovarian-tissue-freezing-better-egg-freezing-420097

21. Moore HC, Unger JM, Phillips KA, Boyle F, Hitre E, Porter D, Francis PA, Goldstein LJ, Gomez HL, Vallejos CS, Partridge AH, Dakhil SR, Garcia AA, Gralow J, Lombard JM, Forbes JF, Martino S, Barlow WE, Fabian CJ, Minasian L, Meyskens FL Jr, Gelber RD, Hortobagyi GN, and Albain KS; POEMS/S0230 Investigators (2015). Goserelin for ovarian protection during breast-cancer adjuvant chemotherapy. New England Journal of Medicine, 372(10):923-932.

22. Nye L, Rademaker A, and Gradishar WJ (2017). Breast cancer outcomes after diagnosis of hormone-positive breast cancer and subsequent pregnancy in the tamoxifen era. Clinical Breast Cancer, 17(4):e185-e189.

23. Oktay K, Hourvitz A, Sahin G, Oktem O, Safro B, Cil A, and Bang H (2006). Letrozole reduces estrogen and gonadotropin exposure in women with breast cancer undergoing ovarian stimulation before chemotherapy. Journal of Clinical Endocrinology and Metabolism, 91(10):3885-3890.

24. Oktay K, Turan V, Bedoschi G, Pacheco FS, and Moy F (2015). Fertility preservation success subsequent to concurrent aromatase inhibitor treatment and ovarian stimulation in women with breast cancer. Journal of Clinical Oncology, 33(22):2424-2429.

25. Pacheco F and Oktay K (2017). Current success and efficiency of autologous ovarian transplantation: A meta- analysis. Reproductive Sciences, 24(8):1111-1120.

26. Peccatori FA, Mangili G, Bergamini A, Filippi F, Martinelli F, Ferrari F, Noli S, Rabaiotti E, Candiani M, and Somigliana E (2017). Fertility preservation in women harboring deleterious BRCA mutations: Ready for prime time? Human Reproduction, 33(2):181-187.

27. Prasath EB, Chan ML, Wong WH, Lim CJ, Tharmalingam MD, Hendricks M, Loh SF, and Chia YN (2014). First pregnancy and live birth resulting from cryopreserved embryos obtained from in vitro matured oocytes after oophorectomy in an ovarian cancer patient. Human Reproduction, 29(2):276-278.

28. Ruddy KJ, Gelber SI, Tamimi RM, Ginsburg ES, Schapira L, Come SE, and Borges VF (2014). Prospective study of fertility concerns and preservation strategies in young women with breast cancer. Journal of Clinical Oncology, 2014; 32:1151–1156.

29. Shandley LM, Spencer JB, Fothergill A, Mertens AC, Manatunga A, Paplomata E, and Howards PP (2017). .Impact of tamoxifen therapy on fertility in breast cancer survivors. Fertility and Sterility, 107(1):243-252.e5.

30. Society for assisted Reproductive Technology (2018). (https://www.sartcorsonline.com/rptCSR_PublicMultYear.aspx?reportingYear=2014.

31. Smitz J, Dolmans MM, Donnez J, Fortune JE, Hovatta O, Jewgenow K, Picton HM, Plancha C, Shea LD, Stouffer RL, Telfer EE, Woodruff TK, and Zelinski MB (2010). Current achievements and future research directions in ovarian tissue culture, in vitro follicle development and transplantation: Implications for fertility preservation. Human Reproduction Update, 16(4):395-414.

32. Uzelac PS, Delaney AA< Christensen GL, Bohler HC, and Nakajima ST (2015). Live birth following in vitro maturation of oocytes retreived from extracorporeal ovarian tissue aspiration and embryo cryopreservation for 5 years. Fertility and Sterility, 104(5):1258-1260.

33. Walter JR, Xu S, Woodruff TK (2017). A call for fertility preservation coverage for breast cancer patients: The cost of consistency. Journal of the National Cancer Institute, 109(5). doi: 10.1093/jnci/djx006.

34. Zavos A and Valachis A (2016). Risk of chemotherapy-induced amenorrhea in patients with breast cancer: A systematic review and meta-analysis. <u>Acta Oncologica</u>, 55(6):664–670.

BREAST CANCER IN PREGNANCY

Frances Wong, M.D. and Michelle Shayne, M.D.

INTRODUCTION

The diagnosis and management of breast cancer in the pregnant patient requires coordinated care between oncology and obstetrics to optimize outcomes for both mother and fetus. An overview of the presentation, management, and prognosis of breast cancer is presented with special issues that need to be taken into account in the pregnant patient. Recommendations are based mostly on retrospective data and case reviews because there are few prospective analyses in this specific population.

EPIDEMIOLOGY

The incidence of pregnancy-associated breast cancer (i.e., diagnosed from nine months before delivery to 12 months after delivery) is estimated at 1 in 3,000-to-10,000 pregnancies, making it the second most common malignancy associated with pregnancy; cervical cancer is the most common. Prevalence increases with maternal age; consequently, the incidence of breast cancers diagnosed during pregnancy is expected to rise with the trend of delayed childbearing (Woo, 2003). Pregnancy at an early age and multiple pregnancies have been shown to have long-term protective effects against breast cancer. In the short-term, however, pregnancy itself can transiently increase the risk of developing breast cancer; this is thought to be secondary to the effects of elevated estrogen and progesterone levels, causing a growth-enhancing effect on premalignant cells (Wohlfahrt, 2001).

The majority of breast cancers diagnosed during pregnancy are poorly differentiated and of advanced stage. This, in part, may be related to delayed diagnosis during pregnancy. As in nonpregnant women, the most common histology is infiltrating ductal carcinoma. Tumors in pregnant women are less often hormone receptor positive (i.e., estrogen receptor or progesterone receptor) compared to tumors in nonpregnant women. The human epidermal growth factor receptor, HER-2/neu, is associated with aggressive malignancies when present in abundance on the cancer cells. Expression of HER-2 has not been well-studied during pregnancy, although a trend toward increased receptor positivity has been reported (Middleton, 2003, and Reed, 2003).

MAKING THE DIAGNOSIS

The diagnosis of breast cancer in women of childbearing age often is prompted by the detection of a mass or thickening of the breast on self-examination or practitioner's examination, but natural breast changes during pregnancy can complicate and delay diagnosis. Breast weight normally doubles in pregnancy, and the increased density and engorgement make clinical examination and a mammogram more difficult to interpret (Scott-Connor, 1995). Also, because most pregnant women have not reached the standard ages at which routine screening mammography is recommended, clinical- or self-examination becomes the sole method of initial detection. Concern for limiting radiation exposure to the developing fetus also may influence patients and practitioners to put off or limit diagnostic imaging, even after a questionable lump is found. Because of these factors, diagnostic delays of one to two months are common. This may adversely affect outcome because a one-month delay in diagnosis can increase the risk of nodal involvement by 1% to 2% (Nettleton, 1996). Thus, index of suspicion should be high for a pregnant woman with a breast mass, and diagnostic workup should not be postponed. Dedicated breast ultrasound is an ideal modality for pregnant women and should be used first. A mass that persists for two to four weeks should be investigated with imaging and biopsied if clinically warranted.

Differential diagnosis of a breast mass includes fibroadenoma, lactating adenoma, cyst, lobular hyperplasia, milk retention cyst, abscess, lipoma, or rarely, a cancer other than breast adenocarcinoma (e.g., lymphoma or sarcoma) (Woo, 2003).

Diagnostic Imaging

Mammography is not contraindicated during any stage of pregnancy, because radiation exposure to the fetus with a standard two-view study is negligible (Nicklas, 2000). The use of an abdominal shield during mammography is recommended, although there have been no dedicated studies comparing the outcomes in cases where shielding was and was not employed.

Ultrasound is an alternative imaging modality that often is used to diagnose breast cancer in pregnant women and should be the first choice imaging test. The ionizing radiation dose in mammography is small, but with ultrasonography, there is no ionizing radiation to elevate concerns for the fetus, as high-frequency sound waves are used to generate imaging. The distinction between various types of masses, including solid masses and cysts, can be made on ultrasound.

Though breast magnetic resonance imaging (MRI) is more sensitive in detecting breast cancer in dense tissue, the effects of MRI on the developing fetus have not been established. The American College of Radiology recommends that an MRI be considered in instances when there is insufficient diagnostic information obtained after other modalities (i.e., mammography and ultrasonography). This is a rare indication for breast MRI and should not be utilized for the initial workup of a palpable abnormality in the breast of a pregnant woman.

The National Radiological Protection Board advises that MRI be avoided in the first trimester, if possible, although this is controversial and based on theoretical considerations. Although not proven to be harmful during human pregnancy, gadolinium contrast tends to be avoided during all stages of pregnancy, because the contrast can cross the placenta and is associated with fetal abnormalities in rats (Shellock, 2004).

Diagnostic Biopsy

The decision of whether or not to biopsy a breast mass is based on clinical examination findings in conjunction with other imaging findings; however, suspicious masses detected on physical examination should be biopsied even if a corresponding mass was not found on mammography. Percutaneous core needle biopsy performed with local anesthesia and using imaging guidance or palpation are the preferred means of tissue sampling at any time during pregnancy. Core needle, incisional, or excisional biopsies have been found to be relatively safe during pregnancy. Local anesthesia is preferred. For masses found within the latter half of the third trimester, postpartum excision is recommended (Collins, 1995).

Staging Evaluation

Staging breast cancer is based on tumor size, the presence and extent of lymph node involvement, and the presence and extent of metastasis outside of the primary breast tumor. Management decisions are based on cancer stage. If locally advanced cancer has been diagnosed (i.e., tumor size greater than 5 cm, presence of four or more involved lymph nodes, or extension to tissues surrounding the breast), or if clinical symptoms are suggestive of involvement of other organs, further imaging is warranted to complete staging and rule out distant metastases. Lung, liver, bone, and brain are the most common areas of distant spread of breast cancer.

If advanced imaging of the chest or abdomen is felt to be indicated during the first trimester, a discussion of the risks and benefits should take place with the patient so she may make an informed decision. Chest evaluation is performed with chest x-ray with abdominal shield. Computed tomography (CT) of the chest usually is avoided during pregnancy due to the large cumulative radiation dose required. If further evaluation is warranted, noncontrast MRI of the thorax is preferred over CT after the first trimester. Evaluation for intra-abdominal or pelvic metastasis can be performed by ultrasound, although it significantly is less sensitive than CT or MRI. As with chest evaluation, CT is not performed during pregnancy, but noncontrast MRI after the first trimester can be considered (Nicklas, 2000, and Shellock, 2004).

In the presence of signs or symptoms suggestive of bone metastases, evaluation can be performed with low-dose radionuclide bone scan, which is reported to be safe during pregnancy (Baker, 1987). Alternatively, noncontrast MRI could be considered after the first trimester. The safety of plain radiographs is unclear. If brain metastases are suspected, noncontrast MRI is the safest and most sensitive mode of imaging.

MANAGEMENT

Breast cancer is treated optimally with multimodality therapy, which may include surgical resection, radiation therapy, and systemic therapy. The standard guidelines for treating women with breast cancer should be applied to treating pregnant patients with a few modifications to ensure safety of the mother and the developing fetus. Delaying therapy on account of pregnancy is not recommended, because the untreated malignancy has the potential to progress, leading to worsened prognosis. Knowing which standard treatments have acceptable safety profiles for use in pregnant patients and which treatments absolutely are contraindicated guides expedient and appropriate therapy.

Prior to starting therapy, a discussion with the patient should allow for weighing the benefits of therapy against the risks of treatment-related toxicities. When a diagnosis of breast cancer is made in the first half of pregnancy, the option of elective termination should be addressed, although patients should be informed that this has not been shown to improve survival outcome (Nubent, 1985, and Clark, 1989).

Locoregional Therapy

Surgical excision is the definitive treatment for eradicating the primary breast tumor and any local spread to surrounding tissues and lymph nodes. Breast and axillary lymph node surgery during any trimester has been associated with minimal fetal risk (Woo, 2003, and Amant, 2010). Breast reconstruction and implant surgery is reserved until after the postpartum period to limit the number of procedures and associated risks.

Full axillary lymph node dissection is warranted if clinically or biopsy-proven positive lymph nodes were detected on diagnosis. Sentinel lymph node biopsy at time of surgery is performed commonly for axillary staging in patients with clinically node-negative breast cancer. However, sentinel lymph node mapping is controversial during pregnancy. The isosulfan blue dye that is used for mapping has been shown to cause skeletal and neurologic effects in rat models. Additionally, potential for allergic/anaphylactic reactions to isosulfan blue dye in the mother can cause harm to the fetus. Because of this, avoiding this agent is recommended in the first trimester. Moreover, there is uncertainty as to whether the lymphatic system is altered in pregnancy, leading to altered axillary mapping results. An alternative mapping procedure, i.e., radiocolloid mapping with technetium-99m, has been shown to be safe in pregnancy and may be used in the first trimester, though this approach may be less accurate than the dye-based approach (Khera, 2008, and Amant, 2010).

In the nonpregnant patient, postoperative radiation therapy is used for further local control in cases where lumpectomy (i.e., wide local excision, also termed breast conserving surgery) was performed (as opposed to a full mastectomy) or in cases of mastectomy that are high risk for local recurrence. The threshold dose of radiation that places increased risk of congenital malformations in pregnant patients has not been determined definitively, but it is believed that the standard doses delivered in localized breast radiation therapy exceed the value considered to be low risk to the fetus. Although recent case reviews have reported successful deliveries following breast radiation during pregnancy, generally, it has been standard practice to recommend delaying radiation therapy until after delivery. If the benefits of radiation therapy are thought to outweigh the risks, however, an informed discussion with the patient should take place. Abdominal shielding during radiation therapy would be essential. Given the limitations of using radiation therapy in pregnancy, mastectomy over breast-conserving therapy is recommended commonly by practitioners and selected by patients (Fenig, 2001, and Woo, 2003).

Systemic Therapy

Systemic therapy is given with the goal of treating the whole body, including areas of potential micrometastases outside of the primary tumor site that are not eradicated with surgical excision. Systemic therapy for breast cancer in nonpregnant women includes chemotherapy, targeted therapy (i.e., trastuzumab, pertuzumab, or neratinib in cases of HER2/neu-positive tumors), and endocrine therapy (i.e., selective estrogen receptor modulators such as tamoxifen or aromatase inhibitors plus chemical ovarian suppression in cases of estrogen- or progesterone-positive tumors). Treatment with targeted therapy is contraindicated in pregnant women due to case reports of serious teratogenic effects (i.e., oligohydramnios, impaired pulmonary development, skeletal abnormalities, and neonatal death) (Bader, 2007, and Witzel, 2008). Since there have been case reports of miscarriage and fetal death with use of tamoxifen, endocrine therapy is contraindicated in pregnancy (Cardonick, 2004). Therefore, the following discussion on systemic therapy focuses on chemotherapy.

Chemotherapy can be used preoperatively (i.e., neoadjuvant treatment) in cases of large-sized tumors to downsize the tumor and facilitate surgical excision. In both early-stage or locally advanced disease, chemotherapy is used postoperatively (i.e., adjuvant treatment) to eradicate micrometastases and thereby reduce risk of recurrence distant from the primary site. In the setting of measurable metastatic disease, systemic therapy becomes the sole method of treatment as a palliative approach to control and contain the disease, reduce symptoms attributable to the cancer, and prolong life.

The available evidence on chemotherapy in the pregnant patient shows that many of the standard agents used in the treatment of breast cancer are relatively safe for both mother and fetus if initiated after the first trimester. The majority of case reports demonstrated uncomplicated live births with low risk of birth defects and low related morbidity in newborns. Standard dosing without need for initial dose adjustment is recommended, but because chemotherapy dosing is based on body surface area, adjustments will be required due to continued weight gain during pregnancy (Giacalone, 1999; Woo, 2003; and Ring, 2005).

The highest teratogenic risk occurs within the first trimester during organogenesis. Risk to the fetus is lower if chemotherapy is delivered in the second and third trimesters, although even at those gestational periods fetal growth restriction, low birthweight, and transient neonatal myeolosuppression can occur (Cardonick, 2004).

Single-agent chemotherapy rarely is used; different classes of medications typically are combined to increase therapeutic response through synergistic effects. Although prospective data are far from extensive, the chemotherapeutic regimens of adriamycin and cyclophosphamide (AC), and fluorouracil, adriamycin and cyclophosphamide (FAC) have been the most studied in pregnancy. In terms of toxicities to the mother or fetus, there have been few major complications noted with either regimen. Thus, either AC or FAC is considered to be standard of care in the pregnant patient (Turchi, 1988; Berry, 1999; and Hahn, 2006). Long-term effects, such as cardiotoxicity in the child or impaired fertility for the woman have been less well studied.

Taxanes (e.g., paclitaxel and docetaxel) are considered among the most active and commonly used chemotherapeutic agents for the management of early stage breast cancer in non-pregnant women. Until recently, data on the safety of this drug class for use in the pregnant patient were sparse. Pregnancy-related changes in chemotherapy pharmacokinetics suggest mechanisms whereby taxane use may have a favorable toxicity profile. P-glycoprotein (Pgp/MDRI/ABCBI), for which taxanes are substrates, is highly expressed on the maternal compartment of the placenta (Mir, 2008). P-glycoprotein protects the fetus from xenobiotics and is thought to possibly decrease transplacental taxane transfer (Anderson, 2005). Docetaxel and paclitaxel, both metabolized by cytochrome P-450 (CYP) 3A4, may have a shorter half-life and higher clearance, since CYP3A4 is significantly increased during the third trimester of pregnancy (Anderson, 2005). One systematic review on the use of taxanes for cancer treatment in the setting of pregnancy evaluated 23 publications describing 40 women and 42 neonates (Mir, 2009). Paclitaxel was used in 21 cases and docetaxel in 16 cases. Both drugs were used in three cases. Of the 40 women studied, 27 had breast cancer. In this study, no spontaneous abortions or intrauterine deaths were observed. Maternal toxicity was of low grade and manageable. One neonate exposed to paclitaxel for management of metastatic breast cancer was born at 32 weeks and developed acute respiratory distress necessitating neonatal intensive care. Possible taxane-related malformation in the form of pyloric stenosis was observed in another neonate whose mother had received doxarubicin, cyclophosphamide, and paclltaxel as well as docetaxel. Overall, this literature review concluded that taxanes during pregnancy demonstrated a favorable toxicity profile when used during the second and third trimesters of pregnancy.

Another review on the use of taxanes for treatment of breast cancer during pregnancy evaluated 16 studies (50 pregnancies) (Zagouri, 2013). Completely healthy neonates were born in 76.7% of cases. The remaining cases showed the following: one neonate born dystrophic and premature, another with mild hydrocephalus, and another with signs consistent with bacterial sepsis. One neonate was hyperbilirubinemic, and another had apnea of prematurity and respiratory distress syndrome. Another neonate had neutropenia and pyloric stenosis. At a median follow-up time of 16 months, 90% of the children were completely healthy, leading the authors of the review to conclude that taxanes may play a potentially promising role.

We use taxanes along with anthracyclines, cyclophosphamide, and fluoropyrimidines at our institution in pregnant patients who also are referred to our high-risk obstetrics and gynecology division.

In the nonpregnant patient, platinum-based regimens (i.e., cisplatin and carboplatin) also are used as a standard treatment in the adjuvant and metastatic setting. These medications are not recommended in the pregnant patient, because increased and unpredictable circulating levels of these medications can occur as a result of decreased albumin levels in the pregnant patient (Zemlickis, 1994). This phenomenon relates to clearing of platinum medications from the body. They are eliminated in the urine when bound to albumin. If circulating albumin is decreased in pregnancy, there is less available for the drug to bind to, leading to decreased clearance of the drug. Serious congenital defects, including hearing impairment, cytopenias, and central nervous system (CNS) abnormalities, have been reported in the newborn (Cardonick, 2004).

Methotrexate is absolutely contraindicated in pregnancy due to delayed clearance and increased risk of fetal anomalies and spontaneous abortion (Ebert, 1997). This agent had been a standard component of older regimens, but it is used less frequently now for breast cancer, having been replaced by newer, more effective agents.

The timing of delivery should be considered in light of the chemotherapy schedule, particularly to avoid potential complications with chemotherapy-related cytopenias. Anemia and thrombocytopenia could lead to bleeding complications with delivery. Neutropenia could lead to increased risk of serious infection for the mother in the peripartum period. Cases of transient neonatal myelosupression also have been reported when chemotherapy was delivered within several days of delivery (Berry, 1999). It is recommended that delivery not be induced during a time when these cell lines are low. In general, chemotherapy should be avoided three to four weeks before delivery. Preterm delivery sometimes is considered to expedite maternal treatment; the risks of prematurity, however, must be weighed against how much difference a delay of two to four weeks in completion of therapy will make for the woman.

Breastfeeding should be avoided while patients are receiving chemotherapy, targeted therapy, or hormonal therapy, because medications are excreted in the breastmilk and can cause toxic effects to the baby (Briggs, 2008). (See the chapter entitled Breastfeeding after Breast Cancer).

Supportive Therapy

There are limited data on the safety and efficacy of agents used to treat nausea and vomiting as pregnant women tend to be excluded from most clinical drug trials. Nonetheless, small clinical trials of pregnant women and case reports offer strategies to address nausea and vomiting of pregnancy. Pyridoxine (vitamin B_6) has been shown to be safe when used during pregnancy but tends to be effective only for mild to moderate cases of nausea. H1 antagonists (i.e., diphenhydramine and meclizine) have few maternal and fetal toxicities, and are considered first-line therapy. The dopamine antagonists prochlorperazine and metoclopramide have been found to be relatively safe. Oral promethazine (both an H1 antagonist and weak dopamine antagonist) also can be considered. Serotonin antagonists (i.e., odensetron and granisetron) can be used in refractory cases (Magee, 2002).

Granulocyte colony stimulating factor (G-CSF) often is given with chemotherapy to aid white blood cell recovery. Therapy with G-CSF has been used safely in pregnancy (Briggs, 2008).

Genetic Testing

Genetic testing is indicated in patients diagnosed with breast cancer under the age of 50 with a strong family history of malignancy or under the age of 40 without necessarily having a significant family history (See the chapter entitled Breast Cancer Genetics.). A positive deleterious gene mutation would affect neither the treatment nor the prognosis, but it would influence surveillance recommendations after primary treatment (i.e., breast MRI along with routine annual mammography), as well as impact decision-making regarding prophylactic bilateral mastectomy or oophorectomy to reduce the risk of developing a second malignancy. These procedures should be discussed with the patient as part of genetic counseling. If a patient chooses further prophylactic surgery, it would take place after delivery and recovery from treatment.

PROGNOSIS

Maternal Outcome

Studies analyzing outcome of pregnant patients with breast cancer have been mixed. While some data show decreased survival in women with breast cancer in pregnancy compared to stage-matched nonpregnant women, other studies show similar survival between pregnant and nonpregnant women matched for age, stage, and other prognostic factors. Studies consistently indicate that there is increased prevalence of more advanced and aggressive disease in pregnant women compared to nonpregnant women of childbearing age, which suggests that delayed diagnosis may play a role. Available data, however, do not support that delayed diagnosis has translated to worsened survival outcome (Zemlickis, 1994; Ibrahim, 2000; and Reed, 2003).

226

Fetal and Neonate Outcome

There have been several reports of breast cancer metastasizing to the placenta and fetus (Tolar, 2003, and Alexander, 2003). Fortunately, these cases are rare, and cancer management during the pregnancy, including surgery and chemotherapy, has led to low related morbidities of newborns (Giacalone, 1999; Hahn, 2006; and Amant, 2010).

CONCLUSION

Because the incidence of breast cancer during pregnancy is expected to rise, as women delay childbearing and their risk of developing breast cancer increases with age, practitioners should have a strong grasp on how to diagnose and manage such patients. Modifications to standard care are aimed at reducing potential toxic effects to the mother and fetus during pregnancy and the peripartum period. An open discussion about the risks and benefits of treatment between the practitioner and the patient will help the patient make informed decisions about her care.

REFERENCES

1. Amant F, Deckers S, Van Calsteren K, Loibl S, Halaska M, Brepoels L, Beijnen J, Carduso F, Gentilini O, Lagae D, Mir O, Neven P, Ottevanger N, Pans S, Peccatori F, Rouzier R, Senn HJ, Struikmans H, Christiaens MR, Cameron D, and Du Bois A (2010). Breast cancer in pregnancy: Recommendations of an international consensus meeting. European Journal of Cancer, 46(18):3158-3168.

2. Anderson GD (2005). Pregnancy-induced changes in pharmacokinetics: A mechanistic-based approach. Clinical Pharmacokinetics, 44(10):989-1008.

3. Antonelli NM, Dotters DJ, Katz VL, and Kuller JA (1996). Cancer in pregnancy: A review of the literature. Part 1. Obstetrical and Gynecological Survey, (1996). 51(2):125-134.

4. Bader AA, Schlembach D, Tamussino KF, Pristauz G, and Pertru E (2007). Anhydramnios associated with administration of trastuzumab and paclitaxel for metastatic breast cancer during pregnancy. The Lancet Oncology, 8(1):79-81.

5. Baker J, Ali A, Groch MW, Fordham E, Economou SG (1987). Bone scanning in pregnant patients with breast carcinoma. Clinical Nuclear Medicine, 12(7):519-524.

6. Berry DL, Theriault RL, Holmes FA, Parisi VM, Booser DJ, Singletary SE, Buzdar AU, and Hortobagyi GN (1999). Management of breast cancer during pregnancy using a standardized protocol. Journal of Clinical Oncology, 17:855-861.

7. Briggs GG (2008). Drugs in Pregnancy and Lactation, (ed. 8). Lippincott Williams & Wilkins, Philadelphia, PA.

8. Cardonick E and Iacobucci A (2004). Use of chemotherapy during human pregnancy. The Lancet Oncology, 5(5):283-291.

9. Clark RM and Chua T (1989). Breast cancer and pregnancy: The ultimate challenge. Clinical Oncology (Royal College of Radiologists), (1):11-18.

10. Collins JC, Liao S, and Wile AG (1995). Surgical management of breast masses in pregnant women. The Journal of Reproductive Medicine, 40(11):785-788.

11. Ebert U, Löffler H, and Kirch W (1997). Cytotoxic therapy and pregnancy. Pharmacology and Therapeutics, 74(2):207-220.

12. Fenig E, Mishaeli M, Kalish Y, and Lishner M (2001). Pregnancy and radiation. Cancer Treatment Reviews, 27;1-7.

13. Giacalone PL, Laffarque F, and Bénos P (1999). Chemotherapy for breast carcinoma during pregnancy: A French national survey. Cancer, 86(11):2266-2272.

14. Hahn K, Johnson PH, Gordon N, Kuerer H, Middleton L, Ramirez M, Yang W, Perkins G, Hortobagyi GN, and Theriault RL (2006). Treatment of pregnant breast cancer patients and outcomes of children exposed to chemotherapy in utero. Cancer, 107:1219-1226.

15. Ibrahim EM, Ezzat AA, Baloush A, Hussain ZH, and Mohammed GH (2000). Pregnancy-associated breast cancer: A case-control study in a young population with a high-fertility rate. Medical Oncology, 2000;17(4):293-300.

16. Khera SY, Kiluk JV, Hasson DM, Meade TL, Meyers MP, Dupont EL, Berman CG, and Cox CE (2008). Pregnancy-associated breast cancer patients can safely undergo lymphatic mapping. The Breast Journal, 14(3):250-254.

17. Magee LA, Mazzotta P, and Koren G (2002). Evidence-based view of safety and effectiveness of pharmacologic therapy for nausea and vomiting of pregnancy. American Journal of Obstetrics and Gynecology, 186(5 Suppl Understanding):S256-261.

18. Middleton LP, Amin M, Gwyn K, Theriault R, and Sahin A (2003). Breast carcinoma in pregnant women: Assessment of clinicopathologic and immunohistochemical features. Cancer, 98(5):1055-1060.

19. Mir O, Berveiller P, Ropert S, Goffinet F, Pons G, Treluyer JM, and Goldwasser F (2008). Emerging therapeutic options for breast cancer chemotherapy during pregnancy. Annals of Oncology, 19(4):607-613.

20. Mir O, Berveiller P, Goffinet F, Treluyer JM, Serreau R, Goldwasser F, and Rouzier R (2010). Taxanes for breast cancer during pregnancy: A systematic review. Annals of Oncology, 21(2):425-426 .

21. Nettleton J, Long J, Kuban D, Wu R, Shaeffler J, and El-Mahdi A (1996). Breast cancer during pregnancy: Quantifying the risk of treatment delay. Obstetrics and Gynecology, 87(3):414-418.

22. Nicklas AH and Baker ME (2000). Imaging strategies in pregnant cancer patients. Seminars in Oncology, 27(6):623-632.

23. Nugent P and O'Connell (1985). Breast cancer and pregnancy. Archives of Surgery. 120(11):1221-1224.

24. Reed W, Hannisdal E, Skovlund E, Thoresen S, Lilleng P, and Nesland JM (2003). Pregnancy and breast cancer: A population-based study. Virchows Archiv, 443(1):44-50.

25. Ring AE, Smith IE, Jones A, Shannon C, Galani E, and Ellis PA (2005). Chemotherapy for breast cancer during pregnancy: An 18-year experience from five London teaching hospitals. Journal of Clinical Oncology, 23(18):4192-4197.

26. Scott-Connor CE and Schorr SJ (1995). The diagnosis and management of breast problems during pregnancy and lactation. American Journal of Surgery, 170(4):401-405.

27. Shellock FG and Crues JV (2004). MR procedures: Biologic effects, safety, and patient care. Radiology, 232(3):635-652.

28. Tolar J and Neglia JP (2003). Transplacental and other routes of cancer transmission between individuals. Journal of Pediatric Hematology/Oncology, 2003;25(6):430-434.

29. Turchi JJ and Villasis C (1988). Anthracyclines in the treatment of malignancy in pregnancy. Cancer, 61(3):435-440.

30. Witzel ID, Müller V, Harps E, Janicke F, and Dewit M (2008). Trastuzumab in pregnancy associated with poor fetal outcome. Annals of Oncology, 19(1):191-192.

31. Wohlfahrt J, Andersen PK, Mouridsen H, and Melbye M (2001). Risk of late-stage breast cancer after a childbirth. American Journal of Epidemiology, 153(11):1079-1084.

32. Woo JC, Yu T, and Hurd TC (2003). Breast cancer in pregnancy: A literature review. Archives of Surgery. 138(1):91-98.

33. Zagouri F, Sergentanis TN, Chrysikos D, Dimitrakakis C, Tsigginou A, Zografos CG, Dimopoulos MA, Papadimitriou CA (2013). Clinical Breast Cancer, 13(1):16-23.

34. Zemlickis D, Klein J, Moselhy G, and Koren G (1994). Cisplatin protein binding in pregnancy and the neonatal period. Medical and Pediatric Oncology, 23(6):476-479.

BREASTFEEDING AFTER BREAST CANCER

Edward R. Newton, M.D., F.B.A.M. and Katrina B. Mitchell, M.D.

Pregnancy and breastfeeding together have represented the complete reproductive model in the healthy development of humans for hundreds of thousands of years. In the last 70 years, humans have attempted to disengage the link between pregnancy and breastfeeding by replacing breastfeeding and breast milk with bottles and artificial breast milk ("ABM" or "formula"). It is not a surprise that artificial breast milk is a very poor substitute for the complex, living, and dynamic fluid designed to support an infant through its highest growth period. A wealth of data (Chowdhury, 2015, and Newton, 2017) demonstrate the health benefits of breastfeeding and breast milk. Breast milk and breastfeeding enhance neurocognitive development, set the foundation and development of innate and adaptive host defenses against pathogens, upregulate and modulate the anti-inflammatory systems, modify the trajectory of somatic and metabolic growth, and, through mother-infant bonding, establish the basis for better socialization and stress reduction. Children and adults accrue higher intelligence quotient (IQ), less infectious disease, less diabetes, less cardiovascular disease, more normal somatic growth, less autoimmune disease, and less cancer. In particular, breastfeeding and breast milk have a dose effect in reducing the risk of breast cancer, especially among BRCA1 mutation carriers and among African-American women with their risk of "triple-negative" breast cancer (Printz, 2015). Breastfeeding and breast milk are the most effective primary prevention behavior.

The Biology of Breastfeeding

Successful breastfeeding requires motivation and persistence, an intact neuroendocrine feedback loop from the nipple-areolar complex to hypothalamus and pituitary, normal release of oxytocin and prolactin, normal erection of the nipple-areolar complex, normal and frequent (ten to 12) nursing episodes per 24 hours, especially night-time nursing, and a supportive environment that reduces the cerebrally mediated inhibition of oxytocin release by the hypothalamus and the posterior pituitary. Additionally, adequate glandular tissue and effective drainage of the mammary gland during nursing are necessary for adequate volume of milk transfer (Newton, 2017). The management and treatment of breast cancer impacts many of these components of success in one or both of the breasts.

Once a healthy pregnancy occurs, the application of breastfeeding support principles will allow successful breastfeeding regardless of whether the new mother is an 18-year-old without breast cancer or a 38-year-old after breast cancer treatment with one normal breast. The guiding principles are creating a positive, caring environment before and after delivery; an educated, motivated, and persistent new mother; application of the known principles of lactation physiology; and careful monitoring for milk transfer between the breastfeeding mother and her infant.

The known physiologic principles in the production of milk are a supply and demand system, the aforementioned feedback loop between the nipple-areolar complex (NAC) and hypothalamic-pituitary axis from which prolactin (anterior pituitary) acts in concert with other hormones to manufacture milk in the alveolar lactocytes. In addition to producing the prolactin, the nipple stimulation feedback loop causes a release of oxytocin from the posterior pituitary. Oxytocin causes the myoepithelial cells that surround the alveolus to contract. The ejection of milk into the lactiferous ducts initiates the second principle of lactation, emptying of the breast. If alveoli and ducts are not emptied for six to eight hours, the lactocytes begin to reduce the manufacture of breast milk. In addition to oxytocin-mediated myoepithelial contractions, milk transfer efficiency is increased greatly by the formation of a functional teat, probably mediated through oxytocin-mediated contraction of muscle cells within NAC. The formation of the teat draws the lactiferous sinuses into the NAC. A specific learned behavior of combined milking, sucking, and swallowing allow the breast milk to be transferred efficiently and the breast is emptied (Weber, 1986).

Early clinical studies (Newton, 1958) confirmed by neuroendocrine evaluation (Uvnas-Moberg, 1997, and Newton, 2017) more recently have established a neuroendocrine feedback loop between the hypothalamus-pituitary axis and the cerebrum. Noxious influences such as pain or psychic stress will inhibit oxytocin release from the posterior pituitary and reduce milk output by 30% to 40%. In addition, oxytocin dampens the stress responses of the hypothalamic-pituitary, i.e., ACTH, epinephrine, and corticosteroids (Uvnas-Moberg, 1997). The excessively stressful experiences of cancer diagnosis and treatment probably play a major role in breastfeeding difficulties. A knowledgeable, caring, and supportive oncology team is a critical component in creating an environment where breastfeeding can be successful. They tell their patient that breastfeeding is a normal part of the reproductive model and verbalize their support for breastfeeding.

The latter short review of the physiology of lactation is very simple for a very complex system. There are several publications and organizations which may help the clinician understand and help with breastfeeding success (Table 1).

Table 1. Useful Resources for Breastfeeding Management

Books	*Breastfeeding Handbook for Physicians*, 2nd Edition, ACOG and AAP publication, 2014
	Breastfeeding: A Guide for the Medical Profession, 8th Edition, Ruth Lawrence and Robert Lawrence, 2016
	Medications in Mothers' Milk, Thomas Hale, 2017
Organizations	Academy of Breastfeeding Medicine
	International Lactation Consultant Association
Journals	Breastfeeding Medicine
	Journal of Human Lactation
Internet	https://www.medsmilk.com
	https://toxnet.nlm.nih.gov

The successful clinical management of breastfeeding occurs prenatally, peripartum, and postpartum. Antepartum education and support help validate the decision, motivation, and persistence through challenges for the prospective mother. Peripartum help and support is promulgated through the guidelines and certification by the Centers for Disease Control and the Baby Friendly Hospital certification. The guidelines include breastfeeding and skin-to-skin contact within 30 to 60 minutes of delivery, on demand breastfeeding at least eight to 12 times per day, including overnight every two to three hours to ensure adequate unilateral supply. The neonate should room-in with mom 23 of 24 hours a day. The neonate should not be supplemented unless a physician orders it. The baby should be monitored closely for an appropriate number of wet diapers (greater than or equal to 6/day), stooling (greater than or equal to 2/day), and weight gain (after four days postpartum, 0.75 to 1 oz/day) (Newton, 2017). If these measures are not met, the dyad should be seen by the breastfeeding support team as soon as possible (within 48 hours) where a supplemental nursing system and/or galactogogues may be considered.

The Challenge to Breastfeed Following Breast Cancer

The diagnosis of breast cancer may be devastating to a woman's health, self-image, and self-confidence, and challenges the uniquely feminine reproductive model. In premenopausal women, the treatment may alter the anatomy of the breast and the hormonal balance for a functioning reproductive model. Pregnancy and breastfeeding after breast cancer add to the challenges and uncertainty of breast cancer diagnosis and treatment.

Breast cancer is the most common cancer in women. In 2014, 236,968 women (123.6 per 100,000 women) were diagnosed with breast cancer (U.S. Cancer Statistics, 1999-2014) and 41,211 died from breast cancer. Between 1999 and 2014, there has been a modest decrease in the incidence of breast cancer (8%) and death rates from breast cancer (23%) per 100,000 women in the United States (U.S.). In 2014, 10% of women newly diagnosed with breast cancer were less than 45 years of age. Figure 1 graphically displays the age-related rates of pregnancy per 1,000 women (Martin, 2017) and incidence of breast cancer per 100,000 women less than 50 years old. The overlap of these curves describes the potential incidence of pregnancy and breastfeeding after diagnosis of breast cancer. Using the number of pregnancies among premenopausal women with a history of breast cancer in the meta-analysis by Valachis (Valachis, 2011), the rate of pregnancy is about 40/1,000 women with a history of breast cancer versus about 100 pregnancies/1,000 women aged 30 to 45 years old without a history of breast cancer (See Figure 1). The analyzed population is limited to pregnancies more than ten months after the diagnosis of breast cancer so as not to add the complicating factor of pregnancy and/or lactation concurrent with active breast cancer and the period of initial therapy for breast cancer.

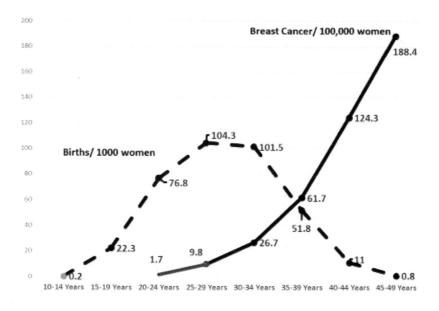

Figure 1. Age-Related Rates of Pregnancy per 1,000 Women and Incidence of Breast Cancer per 100,000 Women Less Than 50 Years Old (Martin, 2017).

Women in resource-rich countries have dramatically changed their motivation and behaviors toward breastfeeding in the last half-century. Since the nadir (27%) in the early 1970s, the initiation of breastfeeding has risen dramatically to better than 81% in 2016 (National Center for Chronic Disease Prevention and Health, 2016, and Newton, 2017). The 2016 breastfeeding initiation rate essentially has met the objective set by the U.S. Surgeon General for Healthy People 2020 for breastfeeding initiation (81%). The duration of exclusive breastfeeding for at least six months and any breastfeeding for 12 or more months (current recommendations) have improved, but they still fall short of the objectives (National Center for Chronic Disease Prevention and Health, 2016). Table 2 depicts the latest U.S. performance versus the Healthy People 2020 Objectives.

Table 2: 2016 United States Breastfeeding Rates versus Healthy People 2020 Objectives.

Behaviors	2020 Objectives	2016 Behaviors
Initiation of Breastfeeding	81.9%	81.1%
Exclusive Breastfeeding for six Months	34.1%	30.7%
Any Breastfeeding at Greater Than or Equal to 12 Months	25.5%	22.3%

Women with a history of breast cancer who desire to become pregnant may have many questions for their healthcare providers. Among the questions are whether they can get pregnant, whether they can produce enough breast milk, would breast milk be safe for their new baby, and will breastfeeding change the prognosis for their breast cancer. Unfortunately, women with a history of breast cancer seem not to breastfeed as often as similar-aged women without a history of breast cancer, 4% versus 10% of women 30 to 45 years old (Figure 1).

Objective study of the incidence and duration of breastfeeding in women with a history of breast cancer is lacking. There are a lack of prospective studies, and the study definitions of breastfeeding are poor. Ideally, measured breastfeeding behaviors should include initiation, exclusivity, duration of breastfeeding, and in the case of mixed feeding, the proportion of feeding that is human milk. In review of the few case series of breastfeeding after breast cancer of ten to 100 cases, the incidence of initiating breastfeeding after breast cancer therapy is 10% to 40%, and the duration is limited to a few weeks. This low rate is despite the presence of a functionally normal breast on the contralateral side. In practice, i.e., twins, one normal breast has the functional capacity to adequately feed one or more infants. For example, one fishing culture in Hong Kong breastfeeds on one breast to facilitate flexibility in bringing in fishing nets. The left to right ratio of breast cancer was 0.97; the left breast was the un-suckled breast. In other populations, the left to right ratio is about 0.50 (Ing, 1977).

Table 3 describes a representative premenopausal population who will face the questions of fertility and breastfeeding. Table 4 describes the variation in treatments in a typical population with breast cancer.

Table 3. A Representative Population of Fertile Women with Breast Cancer

Age at diagnosis	35 to 38 years
Age less than 35 years old	2% to 3%
Primary tumor size greater than or equal to 2 cm	50%
Number lymph nodes positive greater than or equal to 1	50%
Axillary lymph node positive	50%
Grade 3 histology	40% to 50%
Estrogen/progesterone positivity	55% to 65%
HER2 over-expression (positive)	25% to 30%
Triple-negative receptor negative tumor	20% to 25%
Invasive lobular or ductal carcinoma	80%
BRCA 1/2 genotype	10% to 15%

Source: Banz-Jansen C, Heinrichs A, Hedderich M, Waldmann A, Dittmer C, Wedel B, Mebes I, Diedrich K, and Fischer D (2012). Archives of Gynecology and Obstetrics, 286(2):489-493. Gnerlich JL, Deshpande AD, Jeffe DB, Sweet A, White N, and Margenthaler JA (2009). Elevated breast cancer mortality in women younger than age 40 years compared with older women is attributed to poorer survival in early-stage disease. Journal of the American College of Surgeons, 208(3):341-347.

Table 4. Representative Treatments for Fertile Women with Operable Breast Cancer

Breast conserving surgery	50%
Simple mastectomy	45%
Bilateral mastectomy	5%
Radiotherapy	85%
Axillary node sampling	80% to 95%
Chemotherapy for lymph node positivity	85% to 95%
Hormonal therapy	55% to 65%
Anti-HER2 therapy	25% to 30%

Source: Banz-Jansen C, Heinrichs A, Hedderich M, Waldmann A, Dittmer C, Wedel B, Mebes I, Diedrich K, and Fischer D (2012). Archives of Gynecology and Obstetrics, 286(2):489-493. Gnerlich JL, Deshpande AD, Jeffe DB, Sweet A, White N, and Margenthaler JA (2009). Elevated breast cancer mortality in women younger than age 40 years compared with older women is attributed to poorer survival in early-stage disease. Journal of the American College of Surgeons, 208(3):341-347.

Surgery

Breast surgery may impact components of breastfeeding success. The neuroendocrine feedback loop may be disrupted by cutting the efferent and afferent sensory nerves to and from the nipple-areolar complex (referred to as the pedicle, containing the ducts, nerves, and blood vessels). Post-surgical scarring and tethering can prevent the normal erection of the nipple or create difficult latch to a distorted areola. Sutures or incisions in a circumareolar rather than a radial orientation may obstruct major lactiferous ducts and block adequate drainage of intact parenchyma when function is needed. The removal of excessive glandular tissue may reduce milk production from that breast; mastectomy is the extreme of this example.

In the absence of a genetic mutation that increases a patient's future risk of developing a contralateral breast cancer, bilateral mastectomy is not indicated in the average patient. Bilateral mastectomy rates have increased dramatically in recent years, but the American Society of Breast Surgeons (ASBS) issued a position statement in 2016 recommending against contralateral prophylactic mastectomy (CPM) for average-risk women with unilateral breast cancer (Boughey, 2016). Even if a patient does undergo testing that reveals a genetic mutation, National Comprehensive Cancer Network (NCCN) guidelines offer the option of high-risk imaging surveillance (mammogram alternating with breast magnetic resonance imaging [MRI] every six months) versus risk-reducing surgery (NCCN Guidelines, 2017). This allows women who desire to breastfeed to undergo breast conserving treatment (BCT) of the index cancer and preserve the contralateral breast at diagnosis; discussion of prophylactic mastectomy always can be revisited after the completion of pregnancy and lactation.

In the last decade, breast conserving treatment has been evolving from larger "lumpectomy" to where BCT involves removing only a small portion of the breast to clear the margins of cancer and preserving the remainder of the parenchyma for functional and cosmetic purposes. Terminology regarding BCT varies, based on the surgeon preference (training decades ago) and background (surgical oncology fellowship); it may be documented as lumpectomy, partial mastectomy, segmental mastectomy, or wide local excision. Quadrantectomy most often refers to removal of an entire quadrant of a breast. Excisional biopsy may be utilized for removal of benign lesions or pathologic diagnosis of a lesion not amenable to core needle biopsy by radiology. Excisional biopsy also is undertaken for operative sampling of "risk lesions" that may be associated with pre-invasive or invasive cancer and/or with a future risk of cancer development, e.g., atypical ductal hyperplasia, atypical lobular hyperplasia, radial scar, or complex sclerosing lesion.

Regardless of the terminology or nature of the underlying lesion, any BCT procedure involves a small incision on the breast and removal of a breast lesion and limited amount of surrounding parenchyma. Breast-conserving treatment surgical incisions are generally are radial in a Langher's line skin fold, periareolar, or inframammary.

Anatomic studies focusing on nipple areolar complex (NAC) innervation have demonstrated important connections to breast surgeries. While innervation patterns vary significantly among individuals, it generally is agreed upon that the NAC is most commonly innervated by the lateral and anterior cutaneous branches of the 3rd, 4th, and 5th intercostal nerves; the 4th lateral cutaneous branch is the most common anatomic pattern. The nerve travels deeply within the pectoralis fascia, exits through the central breast parenchyma, and reaches the nipple at its posterior surface. In approximately 10% of breasts, the 4th lateral cutaneous branch travels superficially through the subcutaneous tissue to reach the NAC. Additional medial innervation is provided by the 3rd and 4th anterior cutaneous branches, which reach the NAC superficially between the 8:00 and 11:00 position of the left breast and 1:00 and 4:00 position of the right breast (Schlenz, 2000). Therefore, incisions that disrupt the base of the breast or periareolar incisions that disrupt superficial nerve courses or retroareolar innervation and ductal tissue represent the greatest potential to negatively affect future breastfeeding. As long as the skin incision remains greater than 4 cm away from the circumareolar edge, the risk of residual cancer is low (Morimoto, 1985).

Breast-conserving treatment (BCT) for cancer can preserve breast function as long as the nipple-areolar complex is preserved; radiotherapy does more harm to ipsilateral breast function. In the last three decades, improvements in the techniques for breast reduction surgery validate the preservation of the above-described anatomy and preservation of the neuroendocrine feedback loop and breastfeeding success.

Kraut (Kraut, 2017) performed a systematic review of the impact of breast reductive surgery, removal of more than 250 gm of tissue for cosmetic indications, on subsequent breastfeeding success. Breastfeeding success was defined as any breastfeeding for six months. They reviewed the literature using Preferred Reporting Items for Systematic Review and Meta-analysis (PRISMA) methodology. Fifty-one studies met their selection criteria. When the greater than 5 cm diameter sub-areolar pedicle arose from a central or inferior position from the chest wall and was not transected, breastfeeding was more likely to be successful. If the pedicle was transected, i.e., free-nipple transplantation, the median success rate (intra-quartile range [IQR]) was 4% (IQR 0 to 38%); partial-preservation median 75% (IQR 37% to 100%), full-preservation median 100% (IQR 75% to 100%). The removal of more than 600 gm did not seem to affect breastfeeding success if the pedicle was preserved.

One example of breast reduction surgery where the pedicle is preserved is reported by Sinno (Sinno, 2013). He reported a series of 931 breast reduction surgeries at a single hospital using a Moufarrage total posterior pedicle reduction mammoplasty. Of these, 148 women reported breastfeeding after the surgery. The measured breastfeeding outcomes were, 1) the frequency of breastfeeding before and after the surgery in women who had a history of breastfeeding; and 2) the monthly duration of any breastfeeding after the surgery compared to a similar group of women from the general population who had not had breast reduction surgery. In the 75 women who reported having breastfed 49% of their previous children, 55% breastfed their subsequent child after breast reduction surgery. Of the 73 women who had no history of breastfeeding children prior to the surgery, 98% breastfed after surgery. Among all women who breastfed, there was no difference in the duration of breastfeeding compared to the general population who delivered at the hospital: any breastfeeding at one month: 59% versus 67%; at two months: 52% versus 47%; at three months: 42% versus 41%; and at four months: 40% versus 33%.

It should be noted that at the time of BCT, breast surgical oncologists often coordinate with plastic surgeons who may perform unilateral or bilateral mastopexy (breast lift) and/or reduction at the time of index cancer resection. Often, this involves transection of the pedicle. If cancer patients do express interest in this procedure but also desire future breastfeeding, they should be counseled this plastic surgery procedure likely will present challenges with lactation and can be deferred until a later date. If extent of invasive cancer or pre-invasive cancer (ductal carcinoma *in situ*) precludes BCT and requires mastectomy, the patient will not be able to lactate on the side of the affected, surgically removed breast. However, she should be expected to lactate on the contralateral, unaffected breast. Patients should be given additional counseling and support during pregnancy and the immediate postpartum period to ensure adequate nutrition.

Radiation

Breast-conserving treatment (BCT) with postoperative radiation is oncologically equivalent to mastectomy alone, with either treatment approach offering a similar risk of cancer recurrence in the future. Postoperative irradiation reduces the risk of local and regional recurrences from 30% to 40%, to 5% to 7% in ten years (Clarke, 2005, and Darby, 2011). Neoadjuvant chemotherapy may downstage larger tumors and allow more BCT followed by radiation (Kuerer, 2001, and Sun, 2017). Generally, most premenopausal breast cancer patients will receive whole breast radiation with possible addition of boost radiation to the surgical bed and/or nodal field radiation (Buchholz, 2009).

The hallmark result of radiation therapy is cell loss. It, therefore, is expected that an irradiated breast would not function normally. Pathologic studies demonstrate that lobular sclerosis and atrophy are present throughout an irradiated breast (Schnitt, 1984). Additional effects resulting from radiation include impaired nipple-areolar complex pliability, overall breast skin thickening in the radiation field, and changes in vascularity (Mohamed, 2016).

Higgins and Haffty (Higgins, 1994) studied 890 patients who underwent whole breast radiation for breast cancer at a single institution; 11 patients who experienced 13 pregnancies after breast cancer treatment were interviewed. All patients reported minimal breast growth during pregnancy. Four patients lactated in the treated breast: two had minimal milk volume and one of those two breastfed for a total duration of four weeks (unknown duration in the other patient). One had moderately decreased milk volume and breastfed for 16 weeks. Volume was not quantified in the fourth patient, who breastfed for a total duration of 28 weeks, mainly from the contralateral breast. She delivered her child 75 months after completing BCT and radiation. She reported the treated breast nipple did not extend correctly for latch and the baby demonstrated a strong preference for the contralateral breast. She did report spontaneous milk drainage from the treated breast during the total duration of seven months breastfeeding from the untreated breast.

A more recent review by Leal, Stuart, and Carvalho (Leal, 2013) on breast radiation and lactation summarized 13 different studies with a total of 102 patients. Forty-one were able to breastfeed for an average 6.2 weeks. Overall, there was a wide variation of lactation experiences, and no patients were documented to have breastfed longer than 16 weeks. Breastfeeding from the normal contralateral breast was not documented. Despite clear pathologic evidence regarding anatomic and histologic changes to breast parenchyma after radiation therapy, differences in radiation dose, utilization of boost to surgical bed, tumor location, variability in surgical excision also confound the data. In addition, there was variability in whether patients received chemotherapy and/or endocrine therapy, which also can affect breast parenchyma and the ability to lactate effectively.

Despite the confounding methodology as the result of case reports and case series review, there are several consistent observations. Radiation seriously affects breast milk production in a dose-dependent fashion. Once a biologic equivalent dose of about 60 Gy is exceeded, it becomes increasing unlikely that the irradiated breast will produce adequate milk, if at all. The degree of glandular injury is clinically evident prenatally. The normal 50% increase in individual breast size (non-pregnant, 400 gm to pregnant, 600 gm) does not occur. Scarring and tissue sclerosis limit a functional formation (erection) of the nipple-areolar complex with stimulation. However, successful breastfeeding can occur using the non-irradiated contralateral breast.

Only two studies (Green, 1989, and Guix, 2000) have compared the content of breast milk from the irradiated breast to the milk from the contralateral side. In three cases, a detailed observation of the irradiated breast during nursing was performed. The women remarked on the reduced growth in their irradiated breast and a failure to develop a functional teat was noted. Biochemical analysis of breast milk from the irradiated side when compared to breast milk from her non-irradiated contralateral side demonstrated consistently decreased volume, more sodium, decreased phosphate, and decreased liver transaminases (LHD,GOT, GPT). The infants seemed not to like the taste from the irradiated breast, but it is unlikely that the breast milk would cause harm. All three women, using primarily their uninjured contralateral breast, had a prolonged breastfeeding experience.

Accelerated Partial Breast Irradiation (APBI) is increasingly being utilized to provide targeted radiation via a catheter to the surgical bed alone and to reduce the total number of weeks that patients undergo radiation. In selected cases, intraoperative radiation (IORT) also is offered. Theoretically, targeted partial breast radiation will preserve unaffected breast parenchyma and better preserve future ability to lactate. However, APBI and IORT are acceptable only in certain low-risk, node-negative tumor phenotypes, sizes, and patient age groups. It is categorized as cautionary in women less than 40 (Correa, 2017). Aside from oncologic treatment principles and appropriate patient selection, possible fistula formation from the catheter entrance site, mastitis risk, and abscess formation are not clearly documented in any substantial studies at this time.

One additional risk of breast irradiation is the increased risk of a second primary cancer including lung, esophageal, thyroid, and sarcomas. The peak occurrence is about ten to 15 years after the breast radiotherapy. The overall hazard ratio (95th% CI) is 1.51 (1.21 to 1.88) (Grantzau, 2016). This information may be important in the education of a premenopausal woman with breast cancer before she wishes to get pregnant and breastfeed.

Chemotherapy

Adjuvant medical therapy includes cytotoxic chemotherapy, hormonal therapy, and anti-HER2 agents. Due to tumor biology and higher presenting stage, cytotoxic chemotherapy often is recommended in premenopausal breast cancer (Table 5) (Apuri, 2017). Examples of anthracyclines include cyclophosphamide and doxorubicin; hormonal agents include selective estrogen receptor modulators (SERMS) such as tamoxifen (generally used in premenopausal patients) and aromatase inhibitors such as anastrole, letrozole, and exeestane (generally used in post-menopausal patients), leuprolide; and, humanized monoclonal antibodies against the extracellular domain of HER2 include trastuzumab and petuzumab.

Table 5. Adjunctive Medical Therapy for Breast Cancer (Apuri, 2017)

Molecular Character	Percent of Breast Cancer Patients	Agents	Duration
Hormone (E/P) +, HER2 -	60% to 70%	Anthracyclines PLUS Taxanes Hormonal	4 to 6 cycles 4 to 6 cycles Continuous, 5 or 10 years*
HER2 +	15% to 20%	Anthracyclines PLUS Taxanes PLUS Anti-HER2 antibodies	4 to 6 cycles 4 to 6 cycles 4 to 6 cycles
Triple-Negative Tumors	10% to 15% Young African Americans	Anthracyclines PLUS Taxanes	4 to 6 cycles 4 to 6 cycles

Premenopausal breast cancer may present with a palpable mass and nodal positivity rather than a small lesion detected on routine mammographic screening; chemotherapy in the neo-adjuvant or adjuvant setting often is indicated. Due to advances in chemotherapy and anti-HER2 targeted therapy, we often favor neo-adjuvant chemotherapy to provide young patients with early, upfront chemotherapy and downstage a mass to enable breast-conserving therapy (BCT) rather than mastectomy. Once treatment itself has been completed, the effect of chemotherapy on breast parenchyma may be difficult to characterize. The potential toxicity of chemotherapeutic agents in breast milk should not persist, but the chemotherapeutic effect on cell division and proliferation may affect milk production. The studies of the volume and constituents of breast milk several years after chemotherapy and a pregnancy have not been performed. Given the capacity of one breast to produce a large amount of breast milk and the clinical experience of many having successful breastfeeding experiences after breast cancer treatment suggests that this concern is not great.

An additional concern is the risk of anthracycline cardiotoxicity (Sawyer, 2013, and Rehammar, 2017). Higher-risk patients include those with chronic hypertension, hypertension, and obesity. The subclinical cardiomyopathy may manifest as congestive heart failure in a subsequent pregnancy complicated by hypertension and/or preeclampsia.

Breastfeeding Support in a New Mother with a History of Breast Cancer

After breast cancer diagnosis and treatment, pregnancy occurs less often than expected (3% to 5%), and subsequent breastfeeding is even more rarely initiated and its duration reduced. This outcome is despite the presence of a normal contralateral breast, which has the reserve to supply adequate nutrition to meet the needs of the child and meet the Healthy People 2020 Objectives. The reasons for this aberration are many and complex and involve breakdowns in society, care team attitudes, the challenges of the disease processes/treatment, and patient challenges. A major overriding issue is failure of our modern culture to consider breastfeeding as an indispensable part of the reproductive model. A second obstacle is care delivery by individuals rather than a team of experts, which includes a reproductive endocrine and infertility specialist.

SUMMARY

The emotional and physical impact of being diagnosed with breast cancer cannot be overstated. Will this shorten my life? How will my family survive without me? Yet, for those in the reproductive years still desiring pregnancy, additional questions quickly surface. After my treatment, is pregnancy possible? And, if so, can I breastfeed my baby?

Today, advances in surgical techniques and the role of radiation and chemotherapy provide a platform for these discussions. Fortunately, these discussions emanate from a team of care providers. The breast surgeon, plastic surgeon, radiation oncologist, medical oncologist, obstetrician, gynecologist, and lactation consultant all play a fundamental role to provide assistance when that most fearful statement is made, "I am sorry, but you have breast cancer."

REFERENCES

1. Apuri A (2017). Neoadjuvant and adjuvant Therapies for breast cancer. Southern Medical Journal, 110(10):639-642.

2. Boughey JC, Attai DJ, Chen SL, Cody HS, Dietz JR, Feldman SM, Greenberg CC, Kass RB, Landercasper J, Lemaine V, MacNeill F, Song DH, Staley AC, Wilke LG, Willey SC, Yao KA, and Margenthaler JA (2016). Contralateral prophylactic mastectomy statement from the American Society of Breast Surgeons: Data on CPM outcomes and risks. Annals of Surgical Oncology, 23(10):3100-3105.

3. Buchholz TA (2009). Radiation therapy for early-stage breast cancer after breast-conserving surgery. New England Journal of Medicine, 360(1):63-70.

4. Chowdhury R, Sinha1 B, Sankar MJ, Taneja1 S, Bhandari1 N, Rollins N, Bahl R, and Martines J (2015). Breastfeeding and maternal health outcomes: A systematic review and meta-analysis. Acta Pædiatrica, 104(467):96–113.

5. Clarke M, Collins R, Darby S, Davies C, Elphinstone P, Evans V, Godwin J, Gray R, Hicks C, James S, MacKinnon E, McGale P, McHugh T, Peto R, Taylor C, and Wang Y (2005). Effects of radiotherapy and of differences in the extent of surgery for early breast cancer on local recurrence and 15-yearsurvival: An overview of the randomized trials. Lancet; 366(9503):2087-2106.

6. Correa C, Harris EE, Leonardi MC, Smith BD, Taghian AG, Thompson AM, White J, and Harris J (2017). Accelerated partial breast irradiation: Executive summary for an ASTRO evidence-based consensus statement. Practical Radiation Oncology, 7(2):73-79.

7. Darby S, McGale P, Correa C, Taylor C, Arriagada R, Clarke M, Cutter D, Davies C, Ewertz M, Godwin J, Gray R, Pierce L, Whelan T, Wang Y, and Peto R (2011). Effect of radiotherapy after breast-conserving surgery on 10-year recurrence and 15-year breast cancer death: meta-analysis of individual patient data for 10 801 women in 17 randomized trials. The Lancet, 378(9804):1707-1716.

8. Grantzau T and Overgaard J (2016). Risk of second non-breast cancer among patients treated with and without postoperative radiotherapy for primary breast cancer: A systematic review and meta-analysis of population-based studies including 522,739 patients. Radiotherapy and Oncology, 2016, 121: 402–413.

9. Green JP (1989). Post-irradiation lactation. International Journal of Radiation Oncology, Biology and Physics, 17(1):244.

10. Guix B, Tello JI, Finestres F, Palma C, and Martínez A (2000). Lactation after conservative treatment for breast cancer. International Journal of Radiation Oncology, Biology, and Physics, 46(2):515–516.

11. Higgins S and Haffty BG (1994). Pregnancy and lactation after breast-conserving therapy for early stage breast cancer. Cancer, 73(8):2175-2180.

12. Ing R, Petrakis NL, and Ho JH (1977). Unilateral breast-feeding and breast cancer. Lancet, 2(8029):124–127.

13. Kraut RY, Brown E, Korownyk C, Katz LS, Vandermeer B, Babenko O, Gross MS, Campbell S, and Allan GM (2017). The impact of breast reduction surgery on breastfeeding: Systematic review of observational studies. PLoS ONE, 12(10):e0186591.

14. Kuerer HM and Singletary SE (2001). Integration of neoadjuvant chemotherapy and surgery in the treatment of patients with breast carcinoma. Breast Disease, 12:69-81.

15. Leal SC, Stuart SR, and Carvalho HA (2013). Breast Irradiation and Lactation: A Review. Expert Review of Anticancer Therapy, 13(2):159-164.

16. Martin JA, Hamilton BE, Osterman MJK, Driscoll AK, and Mathews TJ (2017) Births: Final Data for 2015 .National Vital Statistics Reports, 66(1):1-70.

17. Mohamed O, McFarlane M, and Rahimi A (2016). Absence of physiologic breast response to pregnancy and lactation. Practical Radiation Oncology, 6(2):e25-6.

18. Morimoto T, Komaki K, Inui K, Umemoto A, Yamamoto H, Harada K, and Inoue K (1985). Involvement of nipple and areola in early breast cancer. Cancer, 1985: 55(10):2459-2463.

19. National Center for Chronic Disease Prevention and Health Promotion, Breastfeeding Report Card Progressing toward National Breastfeeding Goals: USA 2016, https://www.cdc.gov. Accessed 1/18/2018.

20. NCCN Guidelines Version 1.2017: Breast cancer screening and diagnosis.

21. Newton ER (2017). Lactation and breastfeeding (Chapter 24). In: SG Gabbe, JR Niebyl, JL Simpson, MB Landon, HL Galan, ERM Jauniaux, DA Driscoll, V Berghella, and WA Grobman, (Eds.). Obstetrics: Normal and Problem Pregnancies, (Ed. 7). New York: Saunders, 517-549.

22. Newton N and Egli GE (1958). The effect of intranasal administration of oxytocin on the let-down of milk in lactating women. American Journal of Obstetrics and Gynecology, 76(1):103-107.

23. Printz C (2015). Breastfeeding may help prevent aggressive breast cancer in African American women. Cancer, 121(5): 643.

24. Rehammar JC, Jensen MJ, McGale P, Lorenzen EL, Taylor C, Darby SC, Videbæk L, Wang Z, and Ewertz M (2017). Risk ratio of heart disease in relation to radiotherapy and chemotherapy with anthracyclines among 19,464 breast cancer patients in Denmark, 1977–2005. Radiotherapy and Oncology, 123(2):299–305.

25. Sawyer DB (2013). Anthracyclines and heart failure. New England Journal of Medicine, 368(12):1154-1156.

26. Schlenz I, Kuzbari R, Gruber H, and Holle J (2000). The sensitivity of the nipple-areolar complex: An anatomic study. Plastic and Reconstructive Surgery, 105(3):905-909.

27. Schnitt SJ, Connolly MD, Harris JR, and Cohen RB (1984). Radiation-induced changes in the breast. Human Pathology, 15(6):545-550.

28. Sinno H, Botros E, and Moufarrege R (2013). The effects of moufarrege total posterior pedicle reduction mammaplasty on breastfeeding: A review of 931 cases. Aesthetic Surgery Journal, 33(7):1002–1007.

29. Sun Y, Liao M, He L, and Zhu C (2017). Comparison of breast-conserving surgery with mastectomy in locally advanced breast cancer after good response to neoadjuvant chemotherapy: A PRISMA-compliant systematic review and meta-analysis. Medicine, 96:43(1-9).

30. U.S. Cancer Statistics Working Group. United States Cancer Statistics: 1999-2014 Incidence and Mortality Web-based Report. Atlanta: U.S. Department of Health and Human Services, Centers for Disease Control and Prevention and National Cancer Institute; 2017. Available at: www.cdc.gov/uscs. Rate of new cancer cases by Age Group, All Races, Female.

31. Uvnas-Moberg K (1997). Oxytocin linked antistress effects—the relaxation and growth response. Acta Physiologica Scandanavia. Supplementum, 640:38-42.

32. Valachis A, Tsali L, Pesce LC, Polyzos NP, Dimitriadis C, Tsalis K, and Mauri D (2011). Safety of pregnancy after primary breast carcinoma in young women: A meta-analysis to overcome bias of healthy mother effect studies. Obstetrical and Gynecological Survey, 65(12):786-793.

33. Weber F, Woolridge MW, and Baum JD (1986). An ultrasonographic study of the organization of sucking and swallowing by newborn infants. Developmental Medicine and Child Neurology, 28(1):19-24.

REFERENCES AND RELATED READINGS
FOR BRIEF DISCUSSIONS

UNDERSTANDING MENOPAUSE (AT THE MOST BASIC LEVEL)
Harlow SD, Gass M, Hall JE, Lobo R, Maki P, Rebar RW, Sherman S, Sluss PM, and de Villiers TJ (2012). Executive summary of the stages of Reproductive Aging Workshop + 10: Addressing the unfinished agenda of staging reproductive aging. Menopause, 19:1-9.

Matthews KA, Crawford SL, Chae CU, Everson-Rose SA, Sowers MF, Sternfeld B, and Sutton-Tyrrell K (2009). Are changes in cardiovascular disease risk factors in midlife women due to chronological aging or to the menopausal transition? Journal of the American College of Cardiology, 54:2366-2373.

Pfeilschifter J, Koditz R, Pfohl M, and Schatz H (2002). Changes in proinflammatory cytokine activity after menopause. Endocrine Reviews, 23:90-199.

Straub RH (2007). The complex role of estrogens in inflammation. Endocrine Reviews, 28:521-574.

Takao T, Kumagai C, Hisakawa N, Matsumoto R, and Hashimoto K (2005). Effect of 17-B-estradiol on tumor necrosis factor-alpha-induced cytotoxicity in the human peripheral T lymphocyte. Journal of Endocrinology, 184:191-197.

MENOPAUSE OR MENOPAUSE TRANSITION: WHEN DOES THE BIOLOGY BEGIN?
Harlow SD, Gass M, Hall JE, Lobo R, Maki P, Rebar RW, Sherman S, Sluss PM, and de Villiers TJ (2012). Executive summary of the stages of Reproductive Aging Workshop + 10: Addressing the unfinished agenda of staging reproductive aging. Menopause, 19:1-9.

Lobo RA (2008). Metabolic syndrome after menopause and the role of hormones. Maturitas, 60:10-18.

Lovejoy JC, Champagne CM, de Jonge L, Xie H, and Smith SR (2008). Increased visceral fat and decreased energy expenditure during the menopausal transition. International Journal of Obesity, 32:949-958.

Matthews KA, Crawford SL, Chae CU, Everson-Rose SA, Sowers MF, Sternfeld B, and Sutton-Tyrrell K (2009). Are changes in cardiovascular disease risk factors in midlife women due to chronological aging or to the menopausal transition? Journal of the American College of Cardiology, 54:2366-2373.

THE STORY OF ESTROGEN: NOT JUST YOUR MOTHER'S HORMONE Canonico M (2014). Hormone therapy and hemostasis among postmenopausal women: A review. Menopause, 21:753-762.

Canonico M, Plu-Bureau, Lowe GD, and Scarabin P-Y (2008). Hormone replacement and risk of venous thromboembolism in postmenopausal women: Systematic review and meta-analysis. BMJ, 31:1227-1231.

Cushman M (2010). Patch instead of pill: A safer menopausal estrogen? Journal of the American Heart Association: Arteriosclerosis, Thrombosis, and Vascular Biology. 30:136-137.

Gross CG (1998). Claude Bernard and the consistency of the internal environment. The Neuroscientist, 4:380-385.

Shufelt, CL, Merz, CNB, Prentice, RL, Pettinger, MB, Rossouw, JE, Aroda, VR, Kaunitz, AM, Lakshminarayan, K, Martin, LW, Phillips, LS and Manson, JE (2014). Hormone therapy dose, formulation, route of delivery, and risk of cardiovascular events in women: Findings from the Women's Health Initiative Observational Study. Menopause, 21:260-266.

Tara JR (2005). One hundred years of hormones, EMBO Reports, 6:490-496.

Vance DA (20047). Premarin: The intriguing history of a controversial drug. International Journal of Pharaceutical Compounding, 11:282-286.

Watson MC (1935). Observations on the treatment of dysmenorrhea with the placental extract "Emmenin." The Canadian Medical Association Journal, 32:609-614.

WAS THE WOMEN'S HEALTH INITIATIVE GOOD OR BAD FOR WOMEN'S HEALTH? Ochnik, AM, Moore NL, Jankovic-Karasoulos T, Bianco-Miotto T, Ryan NK, Thomas MR, Birrell SN, Burler LM, Tilley WD, and Hickey TE (2013). Antiandrogenic actions of medroxyprogesterone acetate on epithelial cells within normal human breast tissues cultured ex vivo. Menopause, 21:79-88.

Rossouw JE, Manson JE, Kaunitz AM, and Anderson GL (2013). Lessons learned from the women's health initiative trials of menopausal hormone therapy. Obstetrics and Gynecology, 121:172-176.

Simon JA (2014). What if the Women's Health Initiative had used transdermal estradiol and oral progesterone instead? Menopause, a21:769-783.

MENOPAUSE, METABOLISM, AND VISCERAL FAT ACCUMULATION Batra A and Siegmund B (2012). The role of visceral fat. Digestive Diseases, 30:70-74.

Frayn KN (2000). Visceral fat and insulin-resistance-causative or correlative? British Journal of Nutrition, 83:s71-77.

Nielsen S, Guo Z, Johnson CM, Hensrud DD, and Jensen MD (2004). Splanchnic lipolysis in human obesity. Journal of Clinical Investigation, 113:1582-1588.

Kredel LI and Siegmund B (2014). Adipose-tissue and intestinal inflammation-visceral obesity and creeping fat. Frontiers of Immunology, 5:462-473.

Chistiakov DA, Bobryshev YV, Kozarov E, Sobenin IA, and Orekhov AN (2015). Role of gut microbiota in the modulation of atherosclerosis-associated immune response. Frontiers in Microbiology, 6:1-7.

Shuster A, Patlas M, Pinthus JH, and Mourtzakis M (2012). The clinical importance of visceral adiposity: A critical review of methods for visceral adipose tissue analysis. British Journal of Radiology, 85:1-10.

Yki-Jarvinen H (2010). Liver fat in the pathogenesis of insulin resistance and type 2 diabetes. Digestive Diseases, 28(1):203-209.

Klein S (2004). The case of visceral fat: Argument for the defense. Journal of Clinical Investigation, 11:1530-1532.

Lobo RA (2008). Metabolic syndrome after menopause and the role of hormones. Maturitas, 60:10-18.

Hanauer S (2005). Obesity and visceral fat: A growing inflammatory disease. Nature Reviews. Gastroenterology and Hepatology, 2:245.

Kabir M, Catalano KJ, Ananthnarayan S, Kim SP, Van Citters GW, Dea MK, and Bergman RN (2005). Molecular evidence supporting the portal theory: A causative link between visceral adiposity and hepatic insulin resistance. American Journal of Physiology, Endocrinology, and Metabolism, 288:E454E461.

Navarro VM and Kaiser UB (2013). Metabolic influences on neuroendocrine regulation of reproduction. Current Opinion in Endocrinology, Diabetes, and Obesity, 20:335-341.

Di Carlo C, Tommaselli GA, Sammartino A, Bifulco G, Nasti A, and Nappi C (2004). Serum leptin levels and body composition in postmenopausal women: effects of hormone therapy. Menopause, 11:466-473.

Hamdy O, Porramatikul S, and Al-Ozairi E (2006). Metabolic Obesity: The paradox between visceral and subcutaneous fat. Current Diabetes Reviews, 2:1-7.

Lovejoy JC, Champagne CM, deJonge L, Xie H, and Smith SR (2008). Increased visceral fat and decreased energy expenditure during the menopausal transition. International Journal of Obesity, 32:949-958.

Janssen I, Powell LH, Kazlauskaite R, and Dugan SA (2010). Testosterone and visceral fat in midlife women: the Study of Women's Health Across the Nation (SWAN) Fat Patterning Study. Obesity, 18:604-610.

Guthrie JR, Dennerstein L, Taffe JR, Ebeling PR, Randolph JF, Burger HG, and Wark JD (2003). Central abdominal fat and endogenous hormones during the menopausal transition. Fertility and Sterility, 79:1335-1340.

METABOLIC SYNDROME AND THE ROLE OF ESTROGEN

Belfiore A and Malaquarnera R (2011). Insulin Receptor and cancer. Endocrine-Related Cancer, 18:R125-R147.

Beilby J (2004). Definition of metabolic syndrome: Report of the national heart, lung, and blood institute/American Heart Association conference on scientific issues related to definition. Circulation, 109: 433-438.

Bird PJ (2006). Why does fat deposit on the hips and thighs of women and around the stomachs of men? Scientific American, May 15.

Di Carlo C, Tommaselli GA, Sammartino A, Bifulco G, Nasti A, and Nappi C (2004). Serum leptin levels and body composition in postmenopausal women: Effects of hormone therapy. Menopause, 11:466-473.

Hamdy O, Porramatikul S, and Al-Ozairi E (2006). Metabolic Obesity: The paradox between visceral and subcutaneous fat. Current Diabetes Reviews, 2:1-7.

Hilf R (1981). The actions of insulin as a hormonal factor in breast Cancer. Banbury Report, 8:317-337.

Hudis CA andGianni L (2011). Triple-negative breast cancer: An unmet medical need. The Oncologist, 16:1-11.

Kohrt WM (2009). Exercise, weight gain and menopause. Medscape Multispecialty, June 29, 2009.

Lobo RA (2008). Metabolic syndrome after menopause and the role of hormones. Maturitas, 60:10-18.

Lovejoy JC, Champagne CM, de Jonge L, Xie H, and Smith SR (2008). Increased visceral fat and decreased energy expenditure during the menopausal transition. International Journal of Obesity, 32:949-958.

Pollak MN (2007). Insulin, insulin like growth factor, insulin resistance and neoplasm. American Journal of Clinical Nutrition, 86:820s-822s.

Salpeter SR, Walsh JM, Ormiston TM, Greyber E, Buckley NS, and Salpeter EE (2006). Meta-analysis: Effect of hormone-replacement therapy on components of the metabolic syndrome in postmenopausal women. Diabetes Obesity Metabolism, 8:538-554.

Stachowiak G. Pertynski T, and Pertynska-Mapczewska M (2015). Metabolic Disorders in menopause. Przegląd Menopauzalny, 14:59-64.

Suba Z (2014). Triple negative breast cancer risk is defined by the defect in estrogen signaling: Prevention and therapeutic implications. Onco Targets and Therapy, 7:147-167.

WHAT DO WE KNOW ABOUT HOT FLASHES IN MENOPAUSE?

American College of Obstetricians and Gynecologists (2014). ACOG practice bulletin no. 141: Management of Menopausal Symptoms. Obstetrics and Gynecology, 123(1):202-216.

Avis NE, Crawford SL, Greendale G, Bromberger JT, Everson-Rose SA, Gold EB, Hess R, Joffe H, Kravitz HM, Tepper PG, and Thruston RC (2015). Duration of Menopausal Vasomotor Symptoms over the Menopause Transition. Journal of the American Medical Association, 175:531-539.

Butt DA, Lock M, Lewis JE, Ross S, and Moineddin R (2008). Gabapentin for the treatment of menopausal hot flashes: A randomized controlled trial. Menopause, 15:310-318.

Carrol DG (2006). Non hormonal therapies for hot flashes in menopause. American Family Physician, 73:457-464.

Crandall CJ, Tseng C-H, Crawford SL, Thurston RC, Gold EB, Johnston JM, and Greendale GA (2011). Association of menopausal vasomotor symptoms with increased bone turnover during the menopausal transition. Journal of Bone and Mineral Research, 26:840-849.

Freeman EW, Guthrie KA, Caan B, Sternfeld B, Cohen LS, Joffe H, Carpenter JS, Anderson GL, Larson JC, Ensrud KE, Reed SD, Newton KM, Sherman S, Sammel MD, and LaCroix AZ (2011). Efficacy of Escitalopram for hot flashes in healthy menopausal women. Journal of the American Medical Association, 305:267-274.

Freedman RR (2001). Physiology of hot flashes. American Journal of Human Biology, 13:453-464.

Grady D (2015). Management of Menopausal Symptoms. New England Journal of Medicine, 355:2338-2347.

Guthrie KA, LaCroix AZ, Ensrud KE, Joffe H, Newton KM, Reed SD, Caan B, Carpenter JS, Cohen LS, Freeman EW, Larson JC, Manson JE, Rexrode K, Skaar TC, Sternfeld B, and Anderson GL (2015). Pooled analysis of six pharmacologic and nonpharmacologic interventions for vasomotor symptoms. Obstetrics and Gynecology, 126:413-422.

Joffe H, Guthrie KA, LaCroix AZ, Reed SD, Ensrud KE, Manson JE, Newton KM, Freeman EW, Anderson GL, Larson JC, Hunt J, Shifren J, Rexrode KM, Caan B, Sternfeld B, Carpenter JS, and Cohen L (2014). Low-dose estradiol and the serotonin-norepinephrine reuptake inhibitor Venlafaxine for vasomotor symptoms: A randomized clinical trial. Journal of the American Medical Association, 174:1058-1066.

Kaunitz AM and Manson JAE (2015). Failure to treat menopausal symptoms: A disconnect between clinical practice and scientific data. Menopause, 22:687-688.

Morrow PKH, Mattair DN, and Hortobagyi GN (2011). Hot Flashes: A review of pathophysiology and treatment modalities. The Oncologist, 16:16581664.

Nelson HD (2004). Commonly used types of postmenopausal estrogen for treatment of hot flashes. Journal of the American Medical Association, 291:1610-1620.

Pandya KJ, Morrow GR, Roscoe JA, Zhao H, Hickok JT, Pajon E, Sweeney TJ, Banerjee TK, and Flynn PJ (2005). Gabapentin for hot flashes in 420 women with breast cancer: A randomized double-blind placebo-controlled trial. Lancet, 366(9488):818-824.

Pinkerton JAV (2015). Money talks: Untreated hot flashes cost women, the workplace and society. Editorial. Menopause, 22:254-255.

Politi MC, Schleinitz MD, and Col NF (2008). Revising the duration of vasomotor symptoms of menopause: A meta-analysis. Journal of General Internal Medicine, 23:1507-1513.

Sarrel P, Portman D, Lefebvre P, Lafeuille M-H, Grittner AM, Fortier J, Gravel J, Duh MS, and Aupperle PM (2015). Incremental direct and indirect costs of untreated vasomotor symptoms. Menopause, 22:260-266.

Shams T, Firwana B, Habib F, Alshahrani A, Ainouh B, Murad MH, and Ferwana M (2007). SSRIS for hot flashes: A systematic review and metaanalysis of randomized trials. Journal of General Internal Medicine, 29:204213.

Sideras K and Loprinzi C (2010). Nonhormonal management of hot flashes for women on risk reduction therapy. <u>Journal of the National Comprehensive Cancer Network</u>, 8:1171-1179.

Simon JA, Portman DJ, Kaunitz AM, Mekonnen H, Kazempour K, Bhaskar S, and Lippman J (2013). Low-dose paroxetine 7.5 mg for menopausal vasomotor symptoms: two randominzed controlled trials. <u>Menopause</u>, 20:1027-1035.

Thurston RC and Joffe H (2011). Vasomotor symptoms and menopause: Findings from the Study of Women's Health Across the Nation. <u>Obstetrics and Gynecology Clinics of North America</u>, 38:489-501.

DOCTOR, WHY DOES IT HURT DOWN THERE?

Baumgart J, Nilsson K, Evers AS, Kallak, TK, and Poromaa IS (2013). Sexual dysfunction in women on adjuvant endocrine therapy after breast cancer. <u>Menopause</u>, 20:162-168.

Boskey ER, Cone RA, Whaley KJ, and Moench TR (2001). Origins of vaginal acidity: High D/L lactate ratio is consistent with bacteria being the primary source. <u>Human Reproduction</u>, 16:1809-1813.

Editorial Vaginal Dialogues (2014). <u>Menopause</u>, 21:437.

Kendall A, Dowsett M, FolkerdE, and Smith I (2006). Caution: Vaginal estradiol appears to be contraindicated in postmenopausal women on adjuvant aromatase inhibitors. <u>Annals of Oncology</u>, 17:584-587.

Pfeiler G, Glatz C, Königsberg R, Geisendorfer T, Fink-Retter A, Kubista E, Singer CF, and Seifert M (2011). Vaginal estriol to overcome side-effects of aromatase inhibitors in breast cancer patients. <u>Climacteric</u>, 14:339-344.

WHY IS MENOPAUSE MANAGEMENT NOT BETTER UNDERSTOOD BY OB/GYN PROVIDERS?

No references. Personal observations.

INTIMACY AND THE BREAST CANCER SURVIVOR

Course JF, LIndzey J, Grandien K, Gustafsson J-A, and Korach KS (1997). Tissue distribution and quantitative analysis of estrogen receptor-alpha (ER alpha) and estrogen receptor-beta (ER beta) messenger ribonucleic acid in the wild-type and ER alpha knockout mouse. Endocrinology, 138:46134621.

Dew JE, Wren BG, and Eden JA (2003). A cohort study of topical vaginal estrogen therapy in women previously treated for breast cancer. Climacteric, 6:45-52.

Kendall A. Dowsett M, Folkerd E, and Smith I (2006). Caution: Vaginal estradiol appears to be contraindicated in postmenopausal women on adjuvant aromatase inhibitors. Annals of Oncology, 17:584-587.

Labrie F, Archer D, Bouchard C, Fortier M, Cusan L, Gomez JL, Girard G, Baron M, Ayotte N, Moreau M, Dube R, Cote I, Labrie C, Lavoie L, Berger L, Gilbert L, Martel C, and Balser J (2009).Intravaginal dehydroepiandrosterone (Prasterone), a physiological and highly efficient treatment of vaginal atrophy. Menopause, 16:907-922.

Melisko ME, Goldman M, and Rugo HS (2010). Amelioration of sexual adverse effects in the early breast cancer patient. Journal of Cancer Survivorship, 4:247-255.

Tan O, Bradshaw K, and Carr BR (2012). Management of vulvovaginal atrophy-related sexual dysfunction in postmenopausal women. Menopause, 19:109-117.

Witherby S, Johnson J, Demers L, Mount S, Littenberg B, Maclean CK, Wood M, and Muss H (2011). Topical Testosterone for breast cancer patients with vaginal atrophy related to aromatase inhibitors: A phase 1/11 study. The Oncologist, 16:424-431.

ESTROGEN AND BREAST CANCER: A LOVE-HATE RELATIONSHIP

Allen E and Diosy AE (1923). An ovarian hormone; preliminary report on its localization, ex traction and partial purification and action in test animals. Journal of the American Medical Association, 81:819-821.

Beatson GT (1896). On the treatment of inoperable causes of carcinoma of the mammary: Suggestions for a new method of treatment with illustrative cases. Lancet, 2:104.

Dawood S and Cristofanilli M (2007). Endocrine resistance in breast cancer: What really matters? Annals of Oncology, 18:1289-1291.

Haddo WR, Wilkinson JM, Paterson E, and Koller PC (1944). Influence of synthetic estrogens upon advanced malignant disease. BMJ, 2:393.

Haldosen L-A, Zhao C, and Dahlman-Wright K (2013). Estrogen receptor beta in breast cancer. Molecular and Cellular Endocrinology, 382:665-672.

Jordan VC (2014). Another scientific strategy to prevent breast cancer in postmenopausal women by enhancing estrogen-induced apoptosis. Menopause, 10:1160-1164.

Jordan VC and Ford LG (2011). Paradoxical clinical effect of estrogen on breast cancer risk: A "new" biology of estrogen-induced apoptosis. Cancer Prevention Research, 4:633-637.

Labrie F, Luu-The V, Labrie C, Belanger A, Simard J, Lin S-X, and Pelletier G (2003). Endocrine and intracrine sources of androgens in women: Inhibition of breast cancer and other roles of androgens and their precursor dehydroepiandrosterone. Endocrine Reviews, 24:152-182.

Lathrop AEC and Loeb L (1916). Further investigations on the origin of tumors in mice. 111. On the part played by internal secretions in the spontaneous development of tumors. Journal of Cancer Research, 1-19.

Lees JC (1937). The inhibition of growth by 1.2:5.6 Dibenzanthracene and other agents. Quarterly Journal of Experimental Physiology, 27:161-170.

Love RR and Philips J (2002). Oophorectomy for breast cancer: History revisited. Journal of the National Cancer Institute, 94:1433-1434.

Melisko ME, Goldman M, and Rugo H (2010). Amelioration of sexual adverse effects in the early breast cancer patient. Journal of Cancer Survivorship, 4:247-255.

Mense SM, Remotti F, Bhan A, Singh B, El-Tamer M, Kei TK, and Bhat HR (2008). Estrogen-induced breast cancer: Alterations in breast morphology and oxidative stress as a function of estrogen exposure. Toxicology and Applied Pharmacology, 232:78-85.

Obiorah I and Jordan VC (2013). Scientific rationale for postmenopause delay in the use of conjugated equine estrogens among postmenopausal women that causes reduction in breast cancer incidence and mortality. Menopause, 20:372-382.

Osborne CK and Schiff R (2005). Estrogen-receptor biology: Continuing progress and therapeutic implications. Journal of Clinical Oncology, 23:1616-1622.

Writing Group for the Women's Health Initiative Investigators (2002). Risks and Benefits of estrogen plus progestin in healthy postmenopausal women. Journal of the American Medical Association, 288-321.

Yager JD and Davidson NE (2013). Estrogen carcinogenesis in breast cancer. New England Journal of Medicine, 354:270-282.

Yager JD (2000). Endogenous estrogens as carcinogens through metabolic activation. Journal of the National Cancer Institute Monographs, 27:67-73.

Zhang Q, Aft RL, and Gross ML (2008). Estrogen carcinogenesis: Specific identification of estrogen-modified nucleobase in breast tissue from women. Chemical Research in Toxicology, 21:1509-1513.

ARE ALL BREAST CANCERS THE SAME? A PARADOX – ESTROGEN'S RELATIONSHIP TO BREAST CANCER

Allen E and Diosy AE (1923). An ovarian hormone: Preliminary report on its localization, ex traction and partial purification and action in test animals. Journal of the American Medical Association, 81:819.

Beatson GT (1896). On the treatment of inoperable causes of carcinoma of the mammary: Suggestions for a new method of treatment with illustrative cases. Lancet, 2:104.

Belfiore A (2011). Malaguarnera R+. Insulin receptor and cancer. Endocrine-Related Cancer, 18:R125-R147.

Dawood S and Cristofanilli M (2007). Endocrine resistance in breast cancer: What really matters. Annals of Oncology, 18:1289-1291.

Dunn BK, Agurs-Collins T, Browne D, Lubet R, and Johnson KA (2010). Health disparities in breast cancer: Biology meets socioeconomic status. Breast Cancer Research and Treatment, 121:281-292.

Haddo WR, Wilkinson JM, Paterson E, and Koller PC (1944). Influence of synthetic estrogens upon advanced malignant disease. BMJ, 2:393.

Hilf R, Livingston JN, and Crofton DH (1988). Effects of diabetes and sex steroid hormones on insulin receptor tyrosine kinase activity in R3230AC mammary adenocarcinomas. Cancer Research, 48:3742-3750.

Hilf R (1981). The actions of insulin as a hormonal factor in breast cancer. Banbury Report 8 in Hormones and Breast Cancer, Cold Spring Harbor Laboratory. 317-337.

Hudis CA and Gianni L (2011). Triple-negative breast cancer: An unmet medical need. The Oncologist, 16:1-11.

Jordan VC (2014). Another scientific strategy to prevent breast cancer in postmenopausal women by enhancing estrogen-induced apoptosis. Menopause, 10:1160-1164.

Jordan VC and Ford LG (2011). Paradoxical Clinical Effect of Estrogen on Breast Cancer Risk: A "new" biology of estrogen-induced apoptosis. Cancer Prevention Research, 4:633-637.

Lees JC (1937). The inhibition of growth by 1.2:5.6 Dibenzanthracene and other agents. Quarterly Journal of Experimental Physiology, 27:161-170.

Love RR and Philips J (2002). Oophorectomy for breast cancer: History revisited. Journal of the National Cancer Institute, 94:1433-1434.

Maiti B, Kundranda MN, Spiro TP, and Daw HA (2010). The association of metabolic syndrome with triple-negative breast cancer. Breast Cancer Research and Treatment, 121:479-483.

Obiorah I and Jordan VC (2013). Scientific rationale for postmenopause delay in the use of conjugated equine estrogens among postmenopausal women that causes reduction in breast cancer incidence and mortality. Menopause, 20:372-382.

Osborne CK and Schiff R (2005). Estrogen-receptor biology: Continuing progress and therapeutic implications. Journal of Clinical Oncology, 23:1616-1622.

Pollak MN (2007). Insulin, insulin-like growth factors, insulin resistance, and neoplasia. American Journal of Clinical Nutrition, 86:820S-822S.

Suba Z (2014). Triple negative breast cancer risk is defined by the defect in estrogen signaling: Prevention and therapeutic implications. Onco Targets and Therapy, 7:147-167.

Yager JD and Davidson NE (2006). Estrogen carcinogenesis in breast cancer. New England Journal of Medicine, 354:270-282.

Yager JD (2000). Endogenous estrogens as carcinogens through metabolic activation. Journal of the National Cancer Institute. Monographs. 27:67-73.

Zhang Z, Wang J, Tacha DE, Li P, Bremer RE, Chen H, Wei B, Xiao X, Da J, Skinner K, Hicks DG, Bu H. and Tang T (2014). Folate receptor alpha associated with triple-negative breast cancer and poor prognosis. Archives of Pathology and Laboratory Medicine, 138:890-895.

BRCA GENES: PROTECTOR FROM OR CAUSE OF BREAST CANCER?

Brandt-Rauf S, Raveis VH, Drummond NF, Conte JA, and Rothman SM (2006). Ashkenazi Jews and breast cancer: The consequences of linking ethnic identity to genetic disease. American Journal of Public Health, 96:1979-1988.

Deng C-X and Wang RH (2003). Roles of BRCA1 in DNA damage repair-a link between development and cancer. Human Molecular Genetics, 12:R1131123.

Murray RK, Granner DK, Mayes PA, and Rodwell VW (2000). DNA organization, replication, and repair (Chapter 38). In: Harper's Illustrated Biochemistry, (Ed. 22). Stamford: Appleton and Lange, 412-434.

National Cancer Institute. BRCA1 and BRCA2: cancer risk and genetic testing. April 1, 2015.

Yoshida K and Miki Y (2004). Role of BRCA1 and BRCA2 as regulators of DNA repair, transcription, and cell cycle in response to DNA damage. Cancer Science, 95:866-871.

Wu J, Lu L-Y, and Yu X (2010). The role of BRCA1 in DNA damage response. <u>Protein Cell</u>, 1:117-123.

CAN SOME CANCER PATIENTS TAKE HORMONE REPLACEMENT THERAPY?

Bae JM and Kim EH (2015). Hormonal replacement therapy and the risk of lung cancer in women: An adaptive meta-analysis of cohort studies. <u>Journal of Preventive Medicine and Public Health</u>, 48(6):280-286.

Barakat RR, Bundy BN, Spirtos NM, Bell J, and Mannel RS (2006). Randomized double-blind trial versus placebo in stage 1 or 11 endometrial cancer: A Gynecologic Oncology Group Study. <u>Journal of Clinical Oncology</u>, 24(4):587-592.

CDC Centers for Disease Control and Prevention "Cancer among women. Posted 6/16/2016.

Eeles RA, Morden JP, Gore M, Mansi J, Glees J, Wenczl M, Williams C, Kitchener H, Osborne R, Guthrie D, Harper P, and Bliss JM (2015). Adjuvant hormone therapy may improve survival in epithelial ovarian cancer: Results of the AHT Randomized Trial. <u>Journal of Clinical Oncology</u>, 33(35):4138-4144.

Paganini-Hill A (1999). Estrogen replacement therapy and colorectal cancer risk in elderly women. <u>Diseases of the Colon and Rectum</u>, 42(10):1300-1305.

Ploch E (1987). Hormonal replacement therapy in patients after cervical cancer treatment. <u>Gynecologic Oncology</u>, 26(2):169-177.

Slatore CG, Chien JW, Au DH, Satia JA, and White E (2010). Lung cancer and hormone replacement therapy: Association in the Vitamins and Lifestyle Study. <u>Journal of Clinical Oncology</u>, 28(9):1540-1546.

BREAST CANCER: TRAGEDY, FOLLOWED BY DISCOVERY, THEN PLAYED FORWARD

No references.

INDEX

replacement therapy (HRT)

        in breast cancer survivors, 32

        colorectal cancer recurrence and, 32

        endometrial cancer recurrence and, 32

        vs. hormone replacement therapy (HRT) in cancer survivors, 32

        ovarian cancer recurrence and, 32

Estrogen treatment

        breast cancer survivors and, 21

        for painful intercourse, 21

        for vaginal dryness, 21

Estrone (E1), 5

        in Premarin, 6

Fat grafting breast reconstruction, 103-104

Feminine Forever, 8, 19-20, 69

Fertility and breast cancer, 203-216. See also Pregnancy and breast cancer

        fertility preservation prior to cancer treatment, 203-208

        fertility treatment after cancer therapy, 210-212

        ovarian protection during cancer treatment, 208-210

        pregnancy after breast cancer, 212

FFA. *See* Free fatty acids

Fluoxetine, 16

Follicle stimulating hormone (FSH), 10

        during menopause transition, 3

Free fatty acids, 11-12

Free muscle-sparing transverse rectus abdominis myocutaneous flap, 102

Free tissue transfer breast reconstruction, 102-103

FSH. *See* Follicle-stimulating hormone (FSH)

Gabapentin, 16

Ghrelin, 11, 14

Glandular secretions discovery, 5

Glasgow Sleep Effort Scale, 180

Glutathione (GSH), 73